CHAPTER 1

INTRODUCTION

I0482337

1–1. Definition and purpose

The subject matter of this bulletin is hypobaric hypoxia, an environmental stress resulting from ascent to progressively higher terrestrial elevation or altitude. This bulletin defines the threshold altitude at which hypobaric hypoxia becomes functionally and medically significant at 1,200 meters (m) (3,937 feet (ft)) above sea level. Throughout this bulletin, the terms altitude, elevation, hypobaric hypoxia, or hypoxia are considered interchangeable. This bulletin provides guidance to military and civilian health care providers, allied medical personnel, unit commanders and leaders to—

   a. Develop an evidence-based prevention program to protect military personnel from altitude stress and associated adverse health effects.

   b. Understand the physiologic responses and adaptations to altitude (chapter 2).

   c. Implement procedures for managing altitude stress (chapter 3).

   d. Understand the principles and proper use of altitude acclimatization tables (chapter 3).

   e. Understand the physical work performance limitations caused by altitude (chapter 4).

   f. Understand the neuropsychological performance limitations caused by altitude (chapter 5).

   g. Understand the diagnosis and treatment of altitude illness and other medical conditions associated with altitude environments (chapter 6).

   h. Identify the risk factors for altitude illnesses and implement prevention and treatment protocols (chapter 6).

   i. Understand the principles and use of the altitude illness probabilities (chapter 6).

   j. Prevent altitude injuries during training and operational deployments.

   k. Provide background information for reporting and data collection of epidemiological information to note trends and to identify individual, work, and environmental factors that are not adequately controlled by preventive measures and policies.

1–2. References

Required and related publications are listed in appendix A.

1–3. Explanation of abbreviations and terms

The glossary contains a list of abbreviations and terms used in this publication.

> Use of trademarked names does not imply endorsement by the U.S. Army but is intended only to assist in identification of a specific product.

1–4. Roles

a. Unit commander, leaders, and medical personnel, preventive medicine officers, medics and combat lifesavers, Soldiers, and local medical commands will coordinate to implement educational and training programs at all levels in the command based on the principles of this document. They should review all training and operations to make sure adequate planning is made for emergency medical support and altitude illness assessment and management where tactically feasible.

b. Unit commanders and leaders, when appropriate, will—

(1) Integrate the medical officer into all unit staff functions.

(2) Assess training/mission hazards from altitude exposure.

(3) Develop and implement controls for altitude exposure.

(4) Ensure Soldiers are provided adequate training, clothing, shelter, food, and beverages for altitude operations.

(5) Modify physical exertion levels to compensate for effects of increasing altitude.

(6) Ensure planning for all aspects of fluid and food availability.

(7) Modify altitude exposures to provide safe alternative training for individuals or units identified as being at particular risk for altitude casualties.

(8) Initiate a buddy system under altitude conditions and have Soldiers check each other for altitude illness.

(9) Ensure the study of terrain elevations at the deployment site in the advance planning stages, to include location(s) of the lowest elevations for possible altitude treatment activities, as well as the mean and highest elevations at the deployment site to assess impact on physical and cognitive work performances and susceptibility to altitude illness.

(10) Obtain regular real-time weather data and predictions to decrease the risk of cold or heat injury or to provide windows of opportunity for critical military operations.

c. Unit medical personnel or area support medical company staff will—

(1) Understand the commander's intent and mission goals, advise the commander on the potential adverse effects of altitude, and propose practical options for control of altitude exposure.

(2) Assess each component of altitude exposure (condition of the Soldier, elevation, duration of exposure, environmental factors, work load and mission requirements) to plan for the primary prevention of altitude illness by answering the following questions:

(a) What is the altitude and duration of altitude exposure?

(b) What is the altitude acclimatization status of the Soldier?

(c) What work intensity and duration are planned?

(d) Will the Soldier be with a buddy who can assist/watch over him or her to identify and mitigate development of altitude illness?

(3) Estimate the altitude acclimatization status of the unit and provide guidance for regulating physical activities according to the altitude and terrain in the deployment site.

(4) Assist the logistician in estimating water, food, clothing, and shelter requirements.

(5) Develop a casualty evacuation plan to include a means of monitoring patients.

(6) Educate the Soldiers about the steps needed to minimize the risk of altitude illness, to include hydration, nutrition, rest, and avoidance of risk factors (performing intense physical activity and ingesting alcohol and/or drugs or engaging in other forms of substance abuse).

(7) Educate Soldiers in recognizing the signs of impending altitude illness and the basics of buddy aid.

(8) Establish observational checks to detect effects of altitude exposure before illness occurs.

(9) Consider implementation of pharmacotherapy as necessary.

  d. Preventive medicine officers will—

(1) Estimate the incidence of altitude illness and arrange required medical support associated with each course of action.

(2) Integrate the estimates of altitude illness incidence and severity, mission-compatible preventive measures and medical support requirements with the alternatives developed by the command staff.

(3) Become aware of what types of illnesses are being seen at sick call and what medications are being used.

(4) Interview Soldiers diagnosed with altitude illness to describe predisposing conditions and the circumstances surrounding the development.

(5) Use the Tri-Service Reportable Medical Events System to report altitude illness casualties.

(6) Communicate to field activities immediately upon recognition of altitude illness sentinel events and clusters.

  e. Medics and combat lifesavers will support the prevention of altitude illness, recognize and treat altitude illness and implement measures to reduce the risk of additional illness.

  f. Soldiers will—

(1) Be familiar with the causes of altitude illness and the risks of developing the illness.

(2) Know the practical measures they can take to prevent or ameliorate altitude illness.

(3) Become familiar with recognizing the early signs and symptoms of altitude illness.

(4) Use the buddy system to monitor performance and health.

(5) Report to the unit medic/medical officer as soon as possible if they or their buddy develops symptoms of altitude illness.

(6) Maintain adequate physical fitness to deal with the increased physiologic stress of altitude.

(7) Consume adequate food for optimal performance at altitude.

(8) Drink enough fluid to stay adequately hydrated.

(9) Ensure their deployment kits contain an initial supply of sunglasses, sunscreen, lip balm, and skin-care items for high ultraviolet exposure.

(10) Attend altitude illness threat and risk communication briefings and receive appropriate written altitude illness prevention materials well in advance of deployment.

  g. Local medical commands will track altitude illnesses and injuries.

This page intentionally left blank

CHAPTER 2

PHYSIOLOGIC RESPONSES AND ADAPTATIONS TO ALTITUDE

2–1. Altitude stress in military operations

  a. Altitude is the vertical height above sea level of a land mass (for example, Mount Everest) or object (for example, aircraft). With increasing altitude, a decrease in the atmospheric barometric pressure causes a proportional decrease in the partial pressure of oxygen. Ultimately, with increasing altitude the oxygen partial pressure falls to a level at which there are measurable changes in physiological responses, physical and cognitive performance, and the emergence of altitude illness. Based on these measurements, functional definitions of altitude stress have been developed. In this bulletin, altitude stress is defined as terrestrial elevations at or above 1,200 m (3,937 ft). At and above this elevation, the decreased availability of oxygen (that is, hypoxia) in the atmospheric air causes functional impairments and altitude illness. Further demarcations of altitudes above 1,200 m (for example, moderate, high, very high and extreme altitudes) are provided later in this chapter. Throughout this bulletin, the terms altitude, elevation, hypobaric hypoxia, or hypoxia are considered interchangeable. Reference to altitude will be presented in meters, which is the measurement of altitude presented on U.S. military grid maps. Conversions between feet and meters is provided in the glossary.

  b. Soldiers participating in military training and deployments do not often encounter altitude stress. Within the U.S., few military installations are located at altitude (table 2–1). Even at these installations, the area available for maneuvers may be very limited. For example, only the very limited mountainous regions of Fort Irwin are above 1,200 m. Thus, opportunities for training at altitude are limited. Nevertheless, the lack of familiarity and experience with strategies to cope with this unique environment should not be minimized because altitude exposure can deleteriously affect health, mental and physical performance, and morale. U.S. military deployments and operations at altitude have increased as a result of combat operations against military units or terrorist organizations based in high mountainous terrain. A list of countries with geographical elevations above 1,200 m is listed in appendix B. Units preparing for deployments to altitude regions should give strong consideration to scheduling training at altitude prior to deployment.

Table 2–1
Major U.S. military installations located at altitude within the U.S.

Military Installation	State	Altitude (m)
Fort Huachuca	AZ	1,432
USMC MWTC	CA	2,061–3,650
Fort Irwin, NTC[1]	CA	700–1,600
NAWS China Lake[1]	CA	640–2,700
Fort Carson	CO	1,780
Peterson AFB	CO	1,885
Air Force Academy	CO	2,031–2,620
Schriever AFB	CO	1,915
Cheyenne Mountain Air Force Station	CO	1,979
Buckley AFB	CO	1,655
Pohakuloa Training Area	HI	0–2,743
Cannon AFB	NM	1,285
Holloman AFB	NM	1,280
Kirtland AFB	NM	1,632
White Sands Missile Range	NM	1,190–2,000
Hawthorne Army Depot	NV	1,285-2,440
NAS Fallon	NV	1,220
Fort Bliss	TX	1,203
Dugway Proving Ground	UT	1,463
Hill AFB	UT	1,450
Tooele Army Depot	UT	1,500
F.E. Warren AFB	WY	1,876
Notes: [1]Indicates limited terrain above 1,200 m.		

Legend :
USMC=U.S. Marine Corps
MWTC=Mountain Warfare Training Center
NTC=National Training Center
NAWS=Naval Air Weapons Station
AFB=Air Force Base
NAS=Naval Air Station

c. U.S. military operations have been conducted successfully in altitude environments where Soldiers were required to endure the effects of hypoxia and push their physiologic limits (for example, Afghanistan). Nevertheless, the altitude environment can impair many aspects of normal military functioning in the field and, ultimately, the mission. These negative impairments can be minimized with training and experience.

(1) Operational problems often arise in altitude terrain. Mission requirements that demand sustained physical activity are most affected by altitude. Soldiers will fatigue sooner or must reduce their pace and/or lighten their load in order to accomplish many activities.

(2) Many Soldiers may develop altitude illnesses that can produce debilitating symptoms and require medical evacuation.

(3) In most Soldiers altitude induces symptoms, such as shortness of breath and rapid heart rate, that are unrelated to illness or injury. These symptoms can produce unwarranted concerns in Soldiers who are unfamiliar with this environment.

(4) Altitude terrain is frequently steep and rugged which increases the metabolic requirements for many activities, thus raising food and water requirements; yet supply can be difficult, resulting in inadequate nutrition and hydration.

(5) Altitude contributes to increased disease and non-battle injury since sick and injured Soldiers are susceptible to medical complications produced by hypoxia.

(6) Mission requirements that demand sustained physical activity increase the risk of developing altitude sickness.

(7) The steep and rugged terrain common to high elevations increases the risk of sustaining contusions and orthopedic injuries.

(8) Altitude contributes to impaired neuropsychological function and mood changes that may adversely affect the morale of the troops.

d. Military operations in remote altitude locations may have minimal logistical support so troops may find themselves under-equipped for the hostile environmental conditions. Soldiers in these situations must rely on their prior training and strong leadership in altitude acclimatization and illness management. This training can determine whether the mission will succeed or fail with mass casualties. Soldiers in these situations often are not fully prepared and consequently require unit commanders and trainers to actively plan to prevent altitude casualties. Military training exercises, whether initial entry training, special badge qualification training, or military operations training, should be conducted in altitude locations. This will provide an opportunity to teach personnel how to follow appropriate guidelines for successful completion of missions in the rugged terrain and while subject to hypoxia indigenous to the altitude environment.

e. Knowledgeable leadership is essential for training in altitude environments and for successful altitude military operations. Soldiers should have confidence that they can master the environment through the use of preventive measures or at least be cognizant of their limitations. Lessons learned from previous altitude deployments must be shared and emphasized. Leaders must learn their unit's capabilities and manage altitude exposure relative to the provided guidance. Guidance is based on the "average" Soldier, although there is significant individual variability. Supporting medical officers must ensure that the principles of this document are incorporated into the commander's plans and are applied to all phases of training and operations (pre, during, and post).

2–2. Altitude and hypoxemia

a. Decreased availability of oxygen in the atmospheric air (hypobaric hypoxia) is the only environmental stress unique to high terrestrial altitude. It lowers the oxygen supply to body tissues which causes altitude illness and a decline in physical and mental performance often seen in military and civilian personnel operating in high mountain terrain. Hypobaric hypoxia can also interact with other factors in the environment to increase the likelihood of environment-related injuries, or it can exacerbate preexisting medical conditions. Given its widespread effects, a basic understanding of hypobaric hypoxia is essential for medical personnel who support military units operating in high mountain regions.

b. There is a curvilinear reduction in the atmospheric barometric pressure (P_B) with increasing altitude (figure 2–1). In figure 2–1, the P_B is measured in millimeters mercury (mmHg). The exact magnitude of the reduction at any geographic location depends on the combination of elevation, latitude, weather, and season. Generally, within 30° latitude of the equator, the prevailing P_B is higher than predicted by the Standard Atmosphere Model, resulting in a "physiological altitude" that is generally 100–200 m lower than the actual terrestrial altitude. Conversely, the atmospheric prevailing P_B is lower than predicted by the Standard Atmosphere Model as one approaches the Poles (for example, South Pole elevation is 2,837 m, but atmospheric P_B is equivalent to 3,352 m). Table 2–2 shows the relationship between altitude and P_B based on the Standard Atmosphere Model (U.S. Standard Atmosphere 1962). To use the table to estimate altitude from a reported P_B in the U.S., use the "Station Pressure" observations from the National Oceanic and Atmospheric Administration (NOAA), usually reported in inches mercury (inHg). The U.S. Air Force (USAF) weather observations usually report P_B in millibars (mb), the North Atlantic Treaty Organization (NATO) Nations report in either mb or hectopascals (hPa), and medical units with arterial blood gas analyzers usually measure P_B in mmHg.

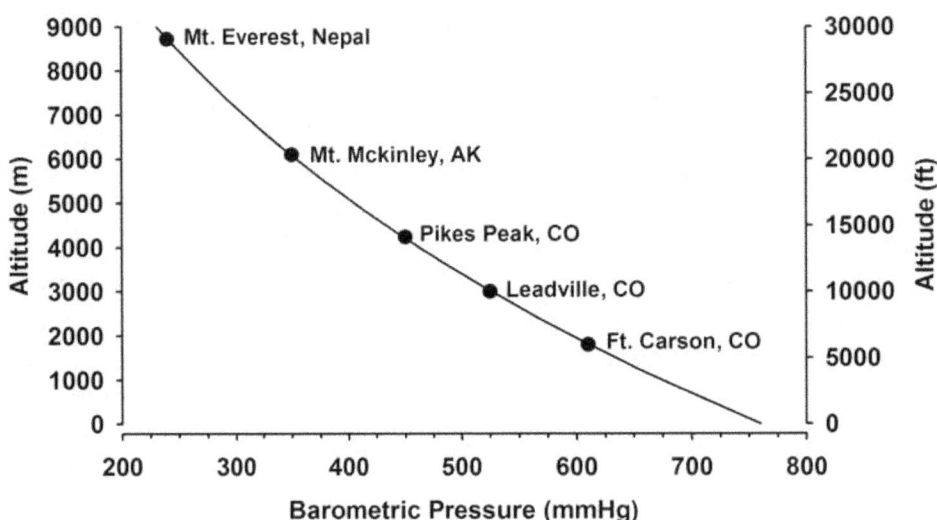

Figure 2–1. Relationship between barometric pressure and increasing altitude

Table 2–2
Relationship between altitude and barometric pressure based on the Standard Atmosphere Model[1]

Altitude (m)	Altitude (ft)	P_B (mmHg)	P_B (inHg)	P_B (mb)	P_B (hPa)
0	0	760	29.92	1013.25	101.32
500	1,641	717	28.23	955.90	95.59
1,000	3,281	674	26.53	898.57	89.86
1,500	4,922	635	25.00	846.58	84.66
2,000	6,562	596	23.46	794.59	79.46
2,500	8,203	561	22.09	747.92	74.79
3,000	9,843	526	20.71	701.26	70.13
3,500	11,484	494	19.45	658.60	65.86
4,000	13,123	462	18.19	615.94	61.59
4,500	14,765	433	17.05	577.27	57.73
5,000	16,405	405	15.94	539.94	53.99
5,500	18,046	380	14.96	506.61	50.66
6,000	19,685	354	13.94	471.95	47.20
6,500	21,327	331	13.03	441.29	44.13
7,000	22,966	308	12.13	410.62	41.06
7,500	24,608	288	11.34	383.96	38.40
8,000	26,247	267	10.51	355.96	35.60
8,500	27,889	249	9.80	331.97	33.20
9,000	29,528	231	9.09	307.97	30.80

Note:
[1]Adapted from U.S. Standard Atmosphere, 1962, U.S. Government Printing Office, Washington, DC, 1962.

c. While the percentage of oxygen (O_2) in one liter of air (that is, 21 percent (%)) does not change at altitude, the partial pressure of O_2 (PO_2) declines with increasing altitude according to Dalton's law of partial pressures ($PO_2 = P_B \times \%O_2$). For example, at sea level the P_B is approximately 760 mmHg, and the PO_2 in atmospheric air is about 160 mmHg (760 mmHg x 0.21). At 5,800 m, P_B is approximately 380 mmHg, and the PO_2 in atmospheric air is only 80 mmHg (380 mmHg x 0.21). As the inspired air passes through the respiratory passages, where it becomes totally saturated with water, the PO_2 is reduced by the partial pressure of water vapor (47 mmHg at body temperature 37 °C). Thus, the PO_2 of moist-inspired gas is given by the expression $PIO_2 = ((P_B-47 \text{ mmHg}) \times 0.21)$. The PO_2 of moist-inspired gas is further reduced in the alveolar air (PAO_2) because of incomplete replacement of alveolar air with atmospheric air, as well as the fact that O_2 is constantly diffusing out of the alveoli into pulmonary capillaries. The PO_2 on the arterial side of the capillary (PaO_2) is slightly less than the PO_2 of alveolar.

Oxygen then rapidly diffuses from the arterial blood into the interstitial tissues and cells of the body. The amount of O_2 extracted by the tissues is proportional to the difference between the PaO_2 and venous O_2 pressure (PvO_2). At each step in the oxygen transport cascade (that is, air to lungs, lungs to blood, blood to tissue), the PO_2 decreases and O_2 flows down its pressure gradient. At altitude, the PO_2 gradient at each level of gas exchange is reduced, and less O_2 is transferred from the environment to the blood as the diffusion of O_2 is directly dependent on the PO_2 gradient (figure 2–2). The result is an impaired ability to transport O_2 to the tissues of the body and the end result is hypoxemia (table 2–3).

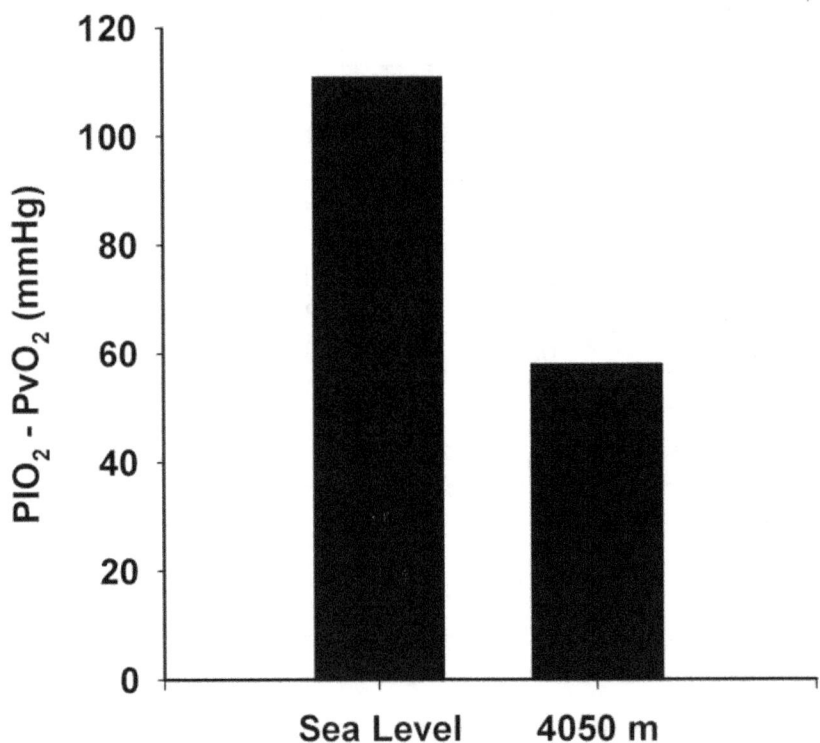

Figure 2–2. Reduction in the oxygen partial pressure gradient from inspired air to venous blood at high altitude compared to low altitude

Table 2–3
Typical acute reductions in the partial pressure of oxygen (O_2) from the atmospheric (PO_2) to inspired (PIO_2), alveolar (PAO_2), arterial blood (PaO_2), and arterial oxyhemoglobin saturation (SaO_2) in resting unacclimatized Soldiers from low to high altitudes

Altitude (m)	PB (mmHg)	PO_2 (mmHg)	PIO_2 (mmHg)	PAO_2 (mmHg)	PaO_2 (mmHg)	SaO_2 (%)
0	760	159	149	104	96	96
1,200	651	138	126	85	74	95
1,600	627	131	121	80	69	94
2,810	543	114	104	65	60	91
3,050	523	110	100	62	58	90
3,660	489	102	93	55	48	85
4,050	463	97	87	49	42	81

d. As stated previously, altitude is defined as elevations at and above 1,200 m. This classification of altitude is based on the relationships between the progressive reduction in arterial PO_2 and the emergence and magnitude of performance decrements, altitude illness and compensatory physiological responses. This classification scheme is presented in figure 2–3. The information presented in figure 2–3 is for unacclimatized low-altitude residents who have rapidly ascended (<6 hours (hr)) from low altitude.

e. The range from sea level up to 1,200 m is considered "low" altitude. In this range, arterial oxyhemoglobin saturation (SaO_2) is generally above 96 percent in healthy people. Also, physiologic changes consistent with altitude acclimatization are absent as is altitude illness and impairments to cognitive performance. Only at the highest range of low altitude is maximal aerobic work performance minimally impaired.

f. "Moderate" altitude extends from 1,200 to 2,400 m (figure 2–3). Generally, resting SaO_2 is normally above 92 percent, and, although the resting SaO_2 is well preserved up to ~2,400 m, the drop in alveolar PO_2 decreases the diffusion of O_2 from the lungs to the blood and then from the blood to the cells. This decrease in O_2 diffusion rate becomes apparent during physical activities as a decrease in SaO_2. Thus, aerobic work performance (for example, a 2-mile run and a 12-mile road march) is decremented at altitudes above 1,200 m, even though resting SaO_2 is near sea-level values. In the moderate altitude range, cognitive performance decrements are not present and altitude illness is very rare. However, the reduced arterial PO_2 is of sufficient magnitude to induce physiological adaptations that are collectively referred to as altitude acclimatization (see paragraph 2–3).

g. "High" altitude extends from 2,400 to 4,000 m. At these elevations, SaO_2 is on the "knee" of the O_2-hemoglobin saturation curve and ranges from approximately 92 to 80 percent (figure 2–3). Aerobic work performance is progressively impaired, and altitude illness and cognitive performance decrements are common in this range of altitude.

h. The region from 4,000 to 5,500 m is classified as "very high" altitude. At altitudes above 4,000 m, the relationship between arterial PO_2 and SaO_2 is on the "steep" portion of the curve where a small decrease in arterial PO_2 results in a relatively large drop in SaO_2 (figure 2–3). Without appropriate altitude acclimatization, Soldiers rapidly ascending from low altitude to very high altitude are at a very high risk of developing debilitating altitude illness and experience very profound impairments of cognitive and physical work performances.

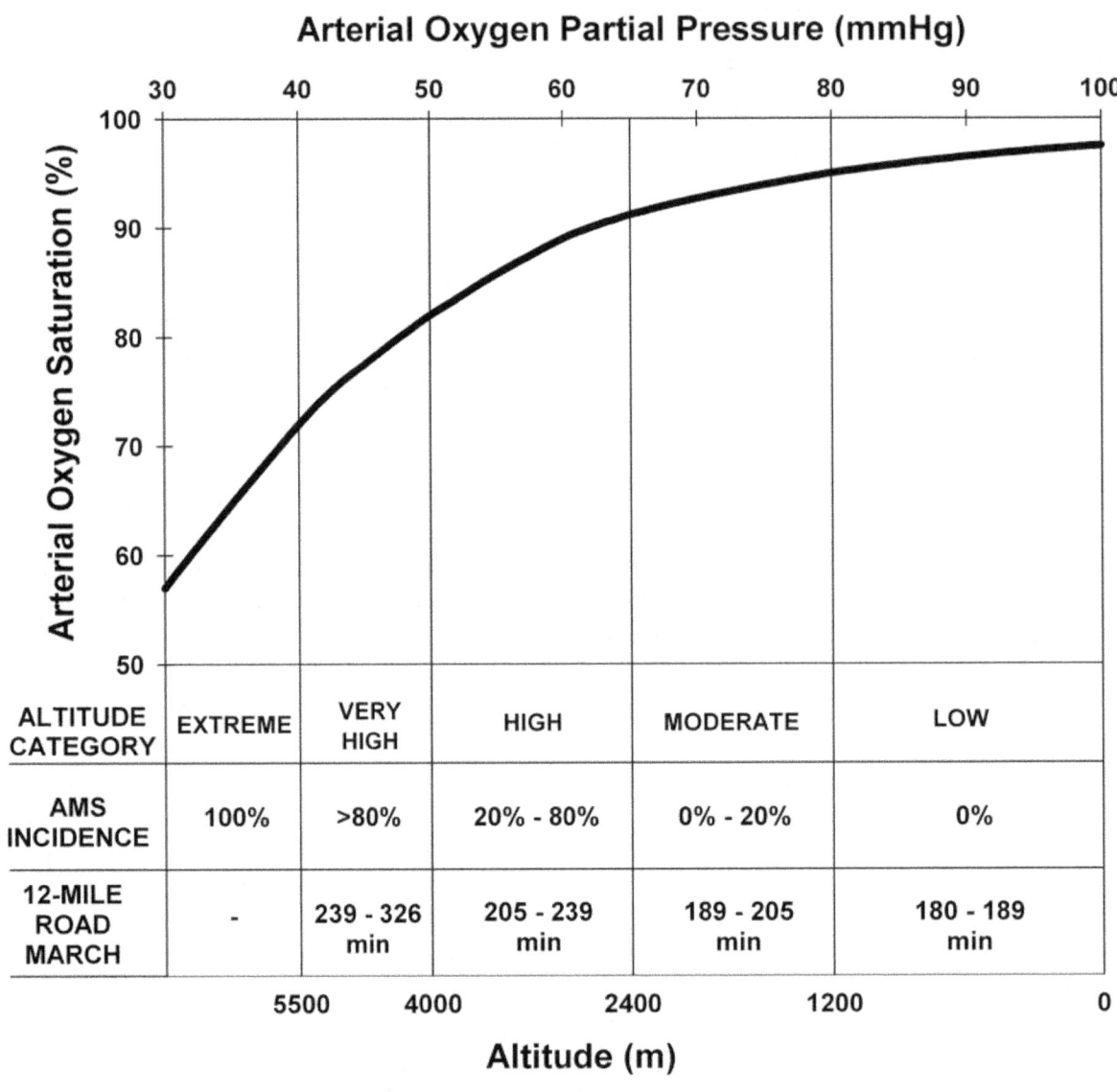

Figure 2–3. Scheme for categorizing altitude based on the relationship between altitude and physiological and functional (work performance and altitude illness) outcomes

i. Altitudes above 5,500 m are classified as "extreme" altitude. Rapid ascent of unacclimatized Soldiers from low altitude to extreme altitude will result in rapid incapacitation and a very high probability of developing potentially fatal altitude illness. While the physiologic adaptations discussed below allow humans to function at extreme altitude for short periods of time, permanent human habitation at these elevations is not possible. In figure 2–3, the upper graph illustrates the relationship among altitude, arterial oxygen partial pressure, and arterial oxygen saturation (SaO_2) in unacclimatized personnel. The information in table format at the bottom of figure 2–3 provides metrics of functional outcomes (aerobic work performance and risk of acute mountain sickness (AMS) as a function of each range of altitudes).

2–3. Adaptations to altitude

a. Exposure to levels of hypoxia inherent to elevations over 1,200 m triggers a series of integrated physiologic changes in Soldiers who ascend from lower altitudes. These changes function to increase O_2 supply to body tissues and are most noticeable in those body systems involved in O_2 delivery (that is, respiratory and cardiovascular), but changes probably occur in all organ systems. Over time, the series of changes produce a state of physiologic adaptation termed "acclimatization." Altitude acclimatization allows Soldiers to achieve the maximum physical and cognitive work performances possible for the altitude to which they are acclimatized. More importantly from a medical perspective, acclimatization is associated with the absence of or very low susceptibility to altitude illness. The rate and success of acclimatization is a function of the interaction between the unique physiologic characteristics of the individual Soldier and the magnitude of hypoxic stress as defined by the elevation gained and the speed of ascent. Acclimatization is elevation-specific, that is full acclimatization to a lower altitude confers only partial acclimatization to a higher altitude (for example, a resident of moderate altitude ascending to high altitude). Once acquired, acclimatization is maintained as long as the Soldier remains at altitude, but is lost over several days to a week or more after return to lower elevations.

> **ALTITUDE STRESS**
> Key Points
> - With increasing altitude, PO_2 decreases (hypoxia).
> - At and above 1,200 meters, hypoxia causes functional impairments and illness.
> - Hypoxia severity increases with altitude.
> - Hypoxia causes physiological adaptations that improve oxygen delivery and utilization.
> - Between 70 and 80 percent of altitude acclimatization occurs in the first week at a specific altitude.
> - Large interindividual variability in physiologic response to hypoxia.

b. The physiologic changes that produce altitude acclimatization affect all phases of oxygen delivery and utilization from gas exchange in the lungs to diffusion of oxygen into mitochondria within individual cells. The major adaptations to altitude are summarized in table 2–4, and the time course of several adaptations and performance metrics is illustrated in figure 2–4. As a general rule, the magnitudes of these physiological adaptations are roughly proportional to the severity of the hypoxic stress, and not all responses are initiated at the same threshold of hypoxia.

Table 2–4
Summary of major physiological adaptations characteristic of altitude acclimatization

Increase Oxygen Delivery	Increase Oxygen Utilization
Increased Ventilation: Raises partial pressure of arterial O_2 (PO_2) and arterial oxyhemoglobin saturation (SaO_2)	Increased Tissue Extraction of O_2 from Capillary Blood
Increased Sympathetic Activity: Sustains blood flow and blood pressure	Increased Carbohydrate Transport and Utilization
Increased 2,3-diphosphoglycerate and Renal Bicarbonate Excretion: Promotes O_2 unloading from hemoglobin	Hypoxia-Inducible Factor (HIF)-Mediated Increased Oxidative Enzyme Function
Decreased Plasma Volume: Raises arterial O_2 content via increased hemoglobin concentration (Hb)	
Erythropoietin Mediated Increase in Red Blood Cell Mass: Raises arterial O_2 content	

   c. Increased ventilation is an immediate response to the reduction in atmospheric PO_2 with increasing altitude. Ventilation increases when the arterial PO_2 is lowered to approximately 70 mmHg or less, a level that is reached at elevations of 1,200 m or greater. Ventilation increases in proportion to the decrease in PO_2 as detected by the peripheral chemoreceptors. The increase in ventilation raises the alveolar and arterial PO_2 by decreasing the partial pressure of alveolar and arterial carbon dioxide. However, the hypoxic-induced hyperventilation causes respiratory alkalosis to develop that in turn blunts the increase in ventilation during the first hours to days of altitude exposure. To compensate for the respiratory alkalosis over the first few days at altitude, increased renal excretion of bicarbonate creates a compensatory metabolic acidosis that sustains and promotes a progressive increase in ventilation, reaching a maximum in 4 to 10 days at a given altitude. Upon further ascent, the process is repeated with further increases in ventilation. Increased ventilation is the principal mechanism responsible for improving the oxygen availability at the cellular level during acclimatization.

d. The onset of hypoxia causes several immediate changes in cardiovascular function. Acute hypoxia decreases PaO_2 and arterial oxygen content which activates the sympathetic nervous system to increase heart rate and systemic blood flow (cardiac output) to maintain systemic O_2 delivery. Although activation of the sympathetic nervous system under a variety of conditions results in peripheral vasoconstriction, local vasodilating mechanisms, responding to the hypoxic stimulus, override sympathetic vasoconstriction and peripheral resistance, and arterial pressure is transiently reduced. In the first 12 hrs of altitude exposure, these disruptions in the maintenance of normal arterial blood pressure can increase the likelihood of orthostatic intolerance, dizziness, and lightheadedness. As O_2 availability increases with altitude acclimatization, the hyperdynamic state of the circulation diminishes, and both cardiac output and peripheral blood flow return toward normal. This decrease in blood flow may be adaptive by allowing more diffusion time for extraction of O_2. Blood pressure gradually rises as the peripheral local mechanisms responsible for vasodilation abate and sympathetic activation continues. Chronic sympathetic hyperactivity, however, leads to down regulation of beta receptors, and a reduction in resting and exercise heart rate occurs with continued altitude exposure. After 3 or more weeks of altitude exposure, stroke volume declines and cardiac output falls below sea-level values. Oxygen uptake is maintained by an increase in O_2 extraction rather than O_2 delivery.

e. During sustained altitude exposure, O_2 delivery to the tissue level is facilitated by a hypoxia-stimulated increase in red blood cell (RBC) 2,3-diphosphoglycerate (2,3-DPG). The increase "shifts" the oxygen-hemoglobin saturation curve to the right, allowing RBCs to release oxygen to the tissues more easily. At high to very high altitudes, the effect is counterbalanced by respiratory alkalosis which tends to shift the curve to the left, making it easier to load O_2 into the RBCs in the lungs and harder to unload it at the tissues. However, at extreme altitudes the effect of the severe respiratory alkalosis predominates, and the curve is shifted to the left. This left shift allows a significant increase in red cell hemoglobin saturation for a given alveolar O_2 pressure at extreme altitude.

f. During altitude exposure, the arterial oxygen content (CaO_2) is increased. Within 12 to 24 hrs of ascent, there is a 5-to-20 percent decrease in plasma volume caused by a movement of fluid out of the vascular compartment into the interstitial and intracellular compartments. In Soldiers who acclimatize normally, this fluid movement produces a diuresis. The magnitude of the plasma volume decrease is proportional to the severity of the hypoxia. The loss of plasma volume produces a relative increase in hemoglobin concentration (Hb) and consequently an increase in effective CaO_2 without an absolute increase in RBC mass. Although erythropoietin (EPO) stimulation occurs within the first hours of altitude exposure, the resultant increase in RBC production is not measurable until 3 or more weeks. During continuous altitude exposure at high to very high altitude, RBC mass may continue to increase for up to 9 months. Plasma volume tends to recover with prolonged (weeks to months) altitude exposure, but the hematocrit and CaO_2 remain high due to the increased RBC mass.

g. Physiological responses to hypoxia involve changes in gene expression that are mediated by the transcriptional activator hypoxia-inducible factor (HIF)-1. Two adaptations increase O_2 utilization by increasing the transport and oxidation of carbohydrates within metabolically active tissues. First, HIF-1 stimulation increases glucose transport across the cell membrane, thus increasing carbohydrate availability within the cell. Second, hypoxic exposure causes an increase in glucose uptake. The preferential use of carbohydrates in a hypoxic environment is supported by the fact that carbohydrates provide the most energy adenosine triphosphate (ATP) per molecule of O_2 transported through the mitochondrial electron transport chain. Thus, in a low O_2 environment, carbohydrates are the best fuel source.

h. Some physiological adaptations to altitude do not appear to be advantageous. In particular, the hypoxic environment causes constriction of the pulmonary arteries raising pulmonary artery pressure. At high to extreme altitudes, the rise in pulmonary artery pressure is great enough to be clinically classified as pulmonary hypertension. The magnitude of the increase in pulmonary artery pressure is to some extent proportional to the magnitude of the hypoxia, and any factors that decrease oxygen levels in the blood tend to exaggerate the increase in pulmonary artery pressure. Such factors include exercise, cold exposure and sleep apnea, all of which are common in Soldiers at high to extreme altitudes. The adaptive function of pulmonary arterial constriction is unclear, but it may improve ventilation/perfusion matching. The hypoxic-mediated increase in pulmonary artery pressure is a contributing factor in the development of high altitude pulmonary edema (HAPE), and may contribute to the decrease in physical work performance (see chapter 4). Cerebral blood flow at altitude is a function of the balance between hypoxia-induced vasodilation and hypocapnia-induced vasoconstriction secondary to hypoxia-induced hyperventilation. Thus, an accentuated hypoxia-induced hyperventilation can cause an acute decrease in cerebral blood flow which, in the presence of hypoxia, can result in loss of consciousness.

i. The sequence of physiologic changes that produce acclimatization to high altitude takes time to complete. The amount of time required for a Soldier to become acclimatized is a function of that individual's physiology and the magnitude of the hypoxic challenge, as defined by the rate of ascent and the altitude attained. At higher altitudes or during fast ascents, the degree of hypoxia is increased, necessitating a more extensive series of physiologic changes that take more time to complete, thus prolonging the time for acclimatization. Soldiers with no recent (>1 month) altitude acclimatization require the greatest physiological compensations and thus the longest time to acclimatize. Soldiers residing at moderate or high altitudes with various degrees of developed acclimatization will achieve acclimatization to a higher altitude more rapidly. At extreme altitude, the degree of hypoxia is so severe that physiologic changes cannot compensate, and Soldiers can never acclimatize completely.

j. For most Soldiers exposed to high and very high altitudes, 70 to 80 percent of the respiratory component of acclimatization occurs in a week to 10 days, and 80 to 90 percent of their overall acclimatization is accomplished by 2 weeks to a month (figure 2-4). Maximum or complete acclimatization may take months to years. While there does not seem to be any way to accelerate all of the physiological processes comprising altitude acclimatization, ventilatory acclimatization can be accelerated by the drug acetazolamide (chapter 6). In figure 2–4, acclimatization outcomes are physical and cognitive performances, AMS, and physiological adjustments (SaO_2 and heart rate).

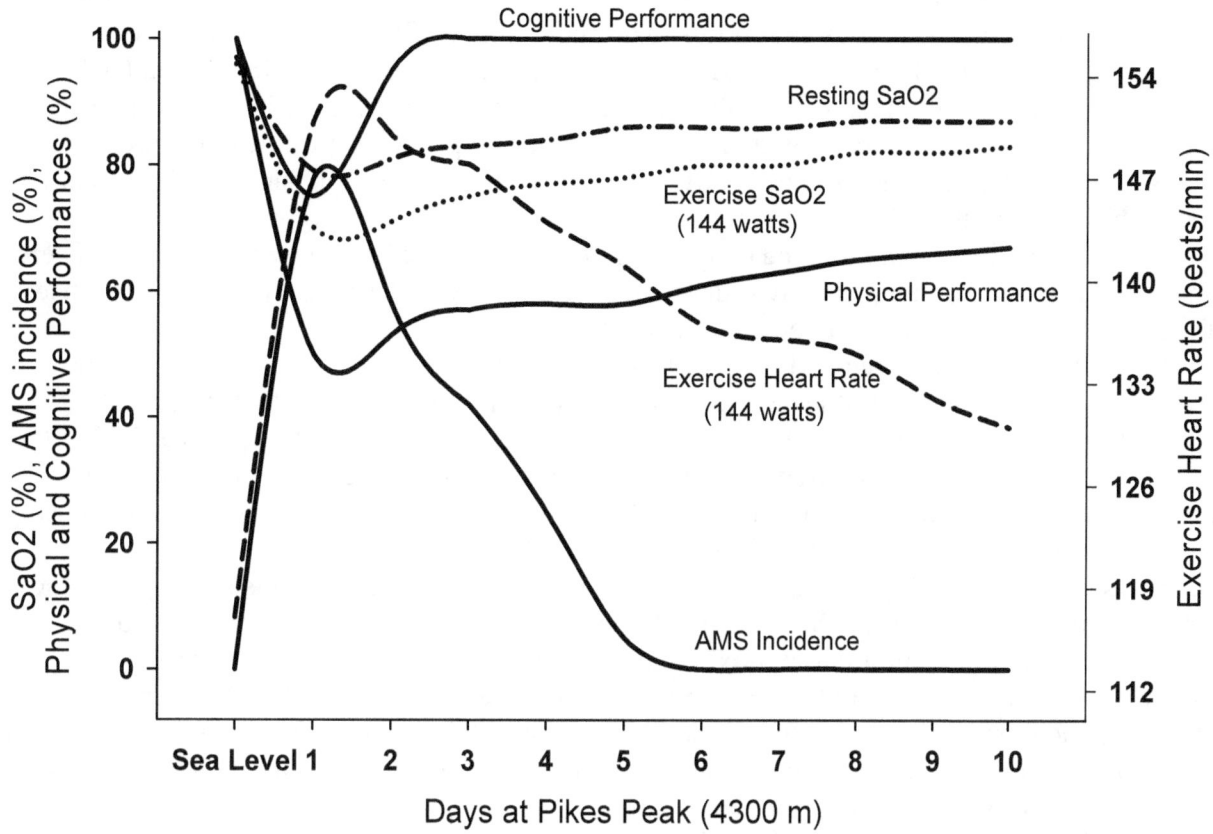

Figure 2–4. Representative time course for altitude acclimatization of low altitude residents directly ascending to 4,300 meters

k. Acclimatization is altitude specific. Once achieved at a given altitude, it will be retained as long as the altitude exposure continues. Exposure to higher altitudes will induce further acclimatization, and descent to lower altitudes will cause a loss of acclimatization, a process often termed "deacclimatization." Acclimatization is probably lost at approximately the same rate or faster than it develops. Soldiers lose 80 to 90 percent of their developed altitude acclimatization in the first 2 weeks of a return to low altitude.

2–4. Individual factors modifying physiological responses to high altitude

a. Currently, no tests can predict individual susceptibility to altitude sickness or the adaptability to altitude of a healthy man or woman residing at low altitudes. Prior histories of altitude sickness or maladaptations to altitude are the best predictors of likely individual responses to future altitude exposures.

b. Some Soldiers acclimatize more rapidly than others. A few individuals appear not to acclimatize at all. Soldiers who do not acclimate can affect unit performance by their own degraded performance and/or as causalities to altitude illness. They should be considered for pharmacotherapy to facilitate acclimatization or a physical profile (Army Regulation (AR) 40-501) to limit their deployment to high altitude areas. Unfortunately, there is no reliable way to identify these individuals except by their experience during previous altitude exposures.

c. Neither gender nor race has been shown to significantly modify physiological responses or susceptibility to altitude illness.

d. There are no known age-related changes in the physiological responses to altitude. There is some evidence that Soldiers who are older than 50 years may be less susceptible to AMS because of the decrease in brain size with advancing age (see chapter 6).

e. Overall, physical training and level of fitness appear to have only minor influences on physiological responses to altitude. Within the range of military fitness standards, greater aerobic fitness does not improve altitude adaptability or decrease susceptibility to altitude illness. However, all Soldiers will experience diminished physical work capacity with increasing altitude, and more fit Soldiers will retain a higher absolute physical work capacity at increasing altitude compared to average fit Soldiers (see chapter 4).

f. The sensitivity of peripheral chemoreceptors and the ventilatory response to hypoxia and carbon dioxide (CO_2) are probably genetically determined and cannot be altered. Soldiers with a decreased ventilatory response to hypoxia may be more susceptible to AMS. Ventilatory response to CO_2 does not seem to be associated with susceptibility to AMS. The sensitivity of peripheral chemoreceptors can be modified by metabolic stimulants such as caffeine and cocoa, respiratory stimulants such as progesterone, respiratory depressants such as alcohol or sleeping medications, and by miscellaneous other factors.

g. Dehydration will increase susceptibility to altitude illness and possibly impair development of altitude acclimatization. Symptoms of dehydration (fatigue, lightheadedness, headache) are similar to symptoms of AMS (see chapter 6). Dehydration may impede the bicarbonate diuresis that compensates for the respiratory alkalosis, thus delaying development of ventilatory acclimatization. Independent from hypoxia, dehydration will impair physical and cognitive work performances.

h. Smoking tobacco increases the percentage of hemoglobin bound to carbon monoxide (CO). This reduces the available hemoglobin for oxygen transport and may exacerbate the hypoxia-induced decrements in physical work performance.

i. Consumption of alcohol can exacerbate the altitude-induced impairments in judgment and the visual senses.

j. Medications that interfere with O_2 transport (ventilation, pulmonary gas exchange, oxyhemoglobin transport, cardiac output, circulation and tissue extraction) or body fluid regulation may impair development of altitude acclimatization and increase susceptibility to altitude illness (see chapter 6).

k. Soldiers with preexisting medical conditions that interfere with O_2 transport or body fluid regulation may be at increased risk for maladaptations to high altitude and increased susceptibility to altitude illness (see chapter 6).

This page intentionally left blank

CHAPTER 3

ALTITUDE RISK MANAGEMENT

3–1. General

  a. Rapid insertion of a military unit into a moderate to extreme altitude environment will cause immediate impairments in physical and cognitive work performance and trigger pathologic conditions collectively referred to as altitude illness. The purpose of this chapter is to provide guidance on recognizing the risks imposed by altitude and implementing effective controls to minimize altitude stress on individual and unit performance and health.

  b. Successful management of altitude stress depends on proper education and experience of leaders and troops exposed to altitude. Successful management of altitude stress results in sustained work capabilities and avoidance of casualties. Composite Risk Management (CRM) is the systematic five-step process of—

  (1) Identifying potential risks.
  (2) Assessing the significance of the risk.
  (3) Developing and selecting controls to minimize the risks.
  (4) Implementing the controls.
  (5) Supervising and evaluating the effectiveness of the controls.

  c. Field Manual (FM) 5–19 recommends using the mission, enemy, terrain and weather, troops and support available, time available, and civil considerations (METT-TC) model to identify potential sources of risk. Leaders must have knowledge and understanding of the risks associated with working in an altitude environment in order to minimize each risk factor imposed by altitude stress.

  d. Table 3–1 lists the most common risk factors that contribute to altitude stress. Using a simplified version of the METT-TC model, there are three principal sources of risk common to operations or training conducted at altitude: environmental, mission, and individual (table 3–1). Most of these risk factors are not unique to the altitude environment. Many impose their own stress on the Soldier independent of the unique altitude stress of hypoxia. However, several of these risks do have specific interactions with hypoxia. These risks factors with known impact on physical and cognitive work performances and susceptibility to altitude illness are listed with their relative impacts (that is, beneficial, no risk, slight risk, moderate risk and significant risk) in table 3–2.

Table 3–1
Risk factors contributing to work performance impairments and medical problems at altitude

Environmental Factors	Mission Factors	Individual Factors
Hypoxia	Ascent Rate	Fitness
Weather	Duration	Nutrition
Solar Radiation	Work Rate	Supplements
Lightning Strikes	Rations	Hydration
Carbon Monoxide		Medication
Terrain		Illness/Injury
		Acclimatization
		Sleep

e. Many independent and related factors will modify the relative impact of a given risk factor in an altitude environment. For example, the risk of an unacclimatized Soldier developing altitude illness following rapid ascent to high altitude varies as a function of altitude exposure duration; that is, the risk is low during the first 6 to 12 hrs, increases between 12 to 48 hrs, and usually decreases to near 0 after 3 to 5 days of exposure. However, continued ascent to increasingly higher altitudes significantly increases the risk of developing altitude illness. Conversely, Soldiers well acclimatized to 2,000 m or higher will be at relatively low risk for developing altitude illness following rapid ascent to altitudes 1,000 to 2,000 m above their acclimatization altitude. Thus, the potential impact of a given risk must be evaluated in the context of total constellation of risks present.

f. Controls can be implemented to minimize many of the risks identified in table 3–2. If an operation must be conducted in an altitude environment, the available controls to minimize the environmental risk factors by themselves are few. However, both individual and mission factors can be modified to reduce the risk imposed by the altitude environment. The most effective control to reduce altitude stress in Soldiers is acquiring altitude acclimatization. A more limited but effective control to reduce susceptibility to altitude illness is pharmaceutical intervention. If possible, one or more of the three mission factors (ascent rate, duration of altitude exposure and work rate) can be modified to reduce the risk of altitude stress. Procedures for inducing altitude acclimatization and/or the use of pharmacotherapies should be included in the operation order medical annex.

Table 3–2
Selected risk factors with known impact on either physical or cognitive work performances at altitude and susceptibility to altitude illness

Risk Factor	Risk Impact		
	Physical Work Performance	**Cognitive Performance**	**Altitude Illness**
Environmental Factors			
Altitude:			
Moderate (1,200–2,400 m)	↓	↔	↓
High (2,400–4,000 m)	↓↓	↓	↓↓
Very High (4,000–5,500 m)	↓↓↓	↓↓↓	↓↓↓
Extreme (>5,500 m)	↓↓↓	↓↓↓	↓↓↓
Cold Temperatures	↔	↔	↓↓
Hot Temperatures	↓↓	↔	↓
Steep and Rugged Terrain	↓	↔	↔
Carbon Monoxide (heaters)	↓↓↓	↓↓↓	↓↓↓
Mission Factors			
Ascent Rate Above 2,400 m:			
>600 m/day	↓↓↓	↓↓↓	↓↓↓
300–600 m/day	↓↓	↔	↓↓
<300 m/day	↓	↑	↓
Duration Above 2,400 m:			
<12 hrs	↓	↓	↔, ↓
12–24 hrs	↓	↔	↓↓↓
1–2 days	↓	↔	↓↓
3–5 days	↓	↑	↓
>5 days	↑	↑	↑
Work Rate:			
Low–Moderate	↓	↔	↓
High–Intense	↓↓	↔	↓↓↓
Individual Factors			
Acclimatized >2,000 m	↑	↑	↑
High Physical Fitness	↑	↔	↔
Adequate Hydration	↑	↑	↑
Nutrition:			
Negative Energy Balance	↓	↓	↓
Increased Carbohydrates	↑	↔	↑, ↔
Preexisting Illness	↔, ↓	↔, ↓	↓
Sleep Deprivation	↓↓	↓↓	↔, ↓

Legend: ↑ = beneficial; ↔ = no risk; ↓ = slight risk; ↓↓ = moderate risk; ↓↓↓ = significant risk

3–2. Altitude acclimatization procedures

   a. General. Altitude acclimatization allows Soldiers to decrease their susceptibility to altitude illness and achieve optimal physical and cognitive performance for the altitude to which they are acclimatized. Altitude acclimatization can be induced in both natural and simulated altitude environments using continuous exposures, such as a staged ascent or graded ascent, and intermittent exposures, such as daily or frequent ascents and descents. Furthermore, altitude acclimatization has no negative side effects and will not harm health or physical performance upon return to low altitude. There are no pharmaceutical therapies that induce altitude acclimatization, but the drug acetazolamide can aid its development (chapter 6). Altitude acclimatization consists of physiological adaptations (chapter 2) that develop in a time-dependent manner during continuous or repeated intermittent exposure to hypoxia. Effective and efficient induction of altitude acclimatization can be accomplished by following two golden rules—

   (1) Ascend to a high enough altitude to create an effective hypoxic stimulus, but not too high that significant altitude illness can develop.

   (2) Reside in the hypoxic environment for a sufficient period of time to allow the adaptations to develop.

   b. Staged ascent. The goal of staged ascent protocols is to promote development of altitude acclimatization while averting the adverse consequences of rapid ascent to higher altitudes (>2,400 m). These staging recommendations will significantly reduce AMS incidence and severity and improve physical and cognitive work performance at higher altitudes.

   (1) Figure 3–1 provides recommended altitude staging profiles between 1,400 and 2,400 m to minimize AMS when ascending another 1,000 to 2,000 m. To use figure 3–1, enter the altitude at which Soldiers will stage (y-axis), then move to the right; when intersecting the dark line, the x-axis provides the exposure duration needed to minimize AMS with further ascent. Altitude staging

---

ALTITUDE ACCLIMATIZATION PROCEDURES
Key Points

- Ascend high enough to induce adaptions, but not so high as to develop altitude illness.
- Unacclimatized Soldiers should *not* ascend above 2,400 m.
- Stage 4–6 days between 2,000–2,400 m.
- Stage 7–14 days between 1,400–2,000 m.
- Staging reduces AMS incidence for altitudes 1,000 to 2,000 m above the staging altitude.
- Graded ascents above 2400 m should not exceed 300 m/day.
- Graded ascents greater than 300 m/day should include a rest day at each higher altitude.

---

requires continuous exposure, and unacclimatized Soldiers should not go beyond 2,400 m without staging. The higher the initial staging altitude, the more quickly altitude acclimatization will be achieved until ~2,400 m; beyond this elevation the risk of developing altitude illness is high, and staging time for unacclimatized Soldiers is at least 3 days. For higher altitudes at or above 3,000 m, the general rule is that staging for 3 or more days will be effective for rapid ascents to 1,000 m above the staging altitude. Staging according to the guidance in figure 3–1 will reduce AMS incidence to 0–10 percent at altitudes up to 3,400 m and to 10–30 percent at altitudes between 3,400–4,400 m. To use, select desired staging altitude, then move to the right to determine the number of staging days required to produce acclimatization. For example, if the staging altitude is 2,000 m, then a minimum of 6 days residence is needed to acquire effective altitude acclimatization.

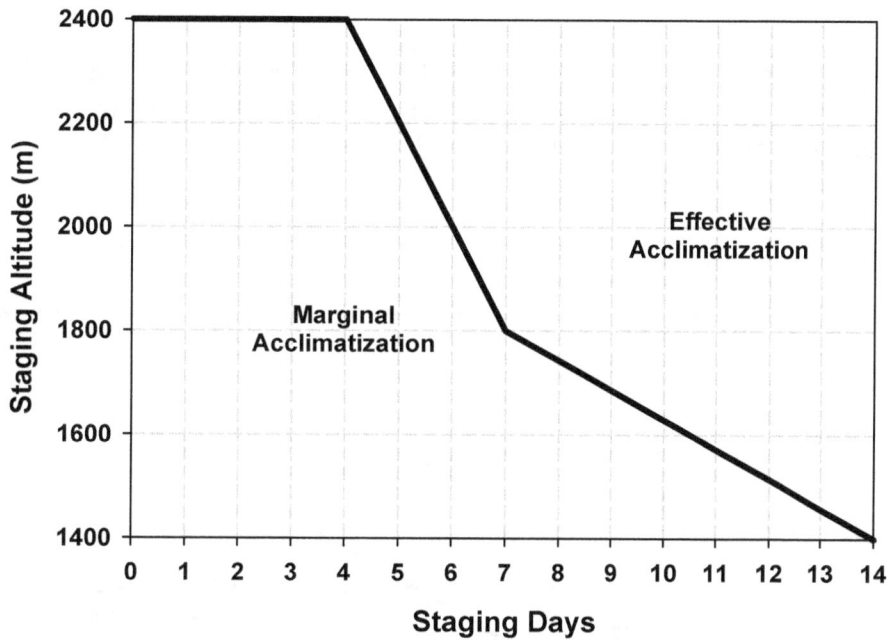

Figure 3–1. Recommended staging altitude and duration combinations to produce effective altitude acclimatization in previously unacclimatized Soldiers

(2) To maximize improvement of physical performance capabilities at altitude, at least 1 hr of moderate-intensity activity (~60 percent maximum heart rate) should be conducted each staging day to promote improved physical performance at that altitude. The greatest physical performance improvements will be attained if the 1-hr aerobic exercise training can be conducted at altitudes at or above 2,000 m.

c. *Graded ascent profiles.* Graded (slow) ascent profiles are a variant of the staging profile and are an option when staging is not possible for unacclimatized personnel ascending to altitudes greater than 2,400 m. Graded ascent profiles are not as effective as altitude staging profiles in reducing AMS incidence and severity above 2,400 m during the first few days of ascent since acclimatization is just developing during this period. Graded ascent profiles are defined as ascents not greater than 600 m per day above 2,400 m. Three examples of graded ascent profiles (150 m/day, 300 m/day and 600 m/day) are illustrated in figure 3–2.

(1) Recommended graded ascent profiles limit the ascent rate to 150–600 m per day and may include a non-ascent day at various intervals. Above 4,000 m, graded ascent profiles should not exceed 300 m over 2 days and should include a non-ascent day every second or third day.

(2) Generally, the slower the ascent above 2,400 m, the lower the risk of developing altitude illness and the better the sustainment of physical and cognitive work performances.

(3) Graded ascent profiles can be used with staging ascent profiles to effectively acclimatize. For example, after using a staged ascent profile from figure 3–1, the acclimatized unit can rapidly ascend to 3,500 m with minimal risk of developing AMS. To ascend above 3,500 m, the unit can use one of the slow ascent profiles in figure 3–2. Personnel rapidly ascending from below 1,200 m should not ascend above 2,400 m for the first night at altitude. Thereafter, one of the three graded ascent profiles should be followed. At altitudes above 4,000 m, daily ascent should not exceed 150 m per day or 300 m every 2 days and should include a non-ascent day every 1 to 2 days.

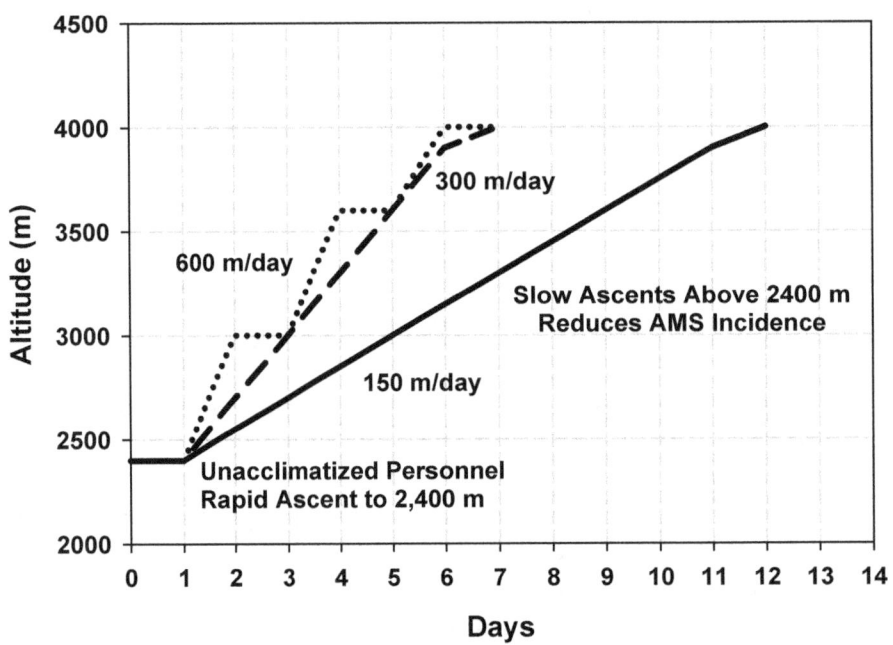

Figure 3–2. Recommended graded ascent profiles to produce effective altitude acclimatization and minimize risk of altitude illness

d. Intermittent altitude (hypoxic) exposure (IHE). A recent approach to inducing altitude acclimatization is the use of repeated, short (less than 24 hrs) altitude or hypoxic exposure in lieu of continuous residence at altitude. Properly conducted intermittent hypoxic exposure can induce altitude acclimatization in personnel residing at low altitudes.

    (1) There are four approaches to producing IHE—

        (a) Natural terrestrial altitude.

        (b) Flight in unpressurized aircraft.

        (c) Flight in pressurized aircraft with high cabin altitudes.

        (d) Normobaric hypoxic devices (nitrogen dilution systems).

    (2) The first three methods of IHE use the natural altitude environment in which barometric pressure is reduced and, thus, may be more effective at inducing altitude acclimatization. Normobaric hypoxia is not as effective as hypobaric hypoxia for inducing altitude acclimatization. Normobaric hypoxic systems are available from commercial sources. All normobaric hypoxic systems have a hypoxic gas source and a means of delivering the hypoxic gas to the user (for example, mask, hood, tent, or room). Advantages of normobaric hypoxic systems are their compact size, portability and ease of operation.

    (3) Guidelines for implementation of IHE conditioning protocols are not well developed. At a minimum, IHE protocols should use altitudes >2,000 m, exposure durations from 3 hrs to as long as possible, and daily exposures, if possible, repeated for a period of at least 1 week or more. Several IHE protocols are presented in table 3–3. Generally, longer daily exposures to altitudes >2,500 m for more than 1 week are more likely to induce functionally useful altitude acclimatization. Soldiers using IHE protocols to induce altitude acclimatization should plan on ascending to altitude as soon as possible after their last IHE.

    (4) When using normobaric hypoxic systems or aircraft in which rapid exposure to hypoxia is possible, the acute exposure to hypoxia may cause lightheadedness and dizziness, particularly at simulated altitudes >3,000 m. Individuals should be aware of this possibility to avoid potential injury. Development of altitude illness during IHE is rare given the usually short exposure duration, but may be present during exposures greater than 4 to 6 hrs.

Table 3–3
Recommended intermittent hypoxic exposure procedures to induce altitude acclimatization in personnel based at low altitude[1]

Session Duration (hrs)	Days	Frequency	Altitude (m)	Activity
3–4	7–14	daily	4,000–4,500	Rest, may include exercise at 50–60% maximum heart rate
>7	>5	daily	2,500–4,000	Rest, sleep, may include exercise at 50–60% maximum heart rate
Note: [1]To avoid sleep disturbances, the first 1–2 nights should not exceed 2,500 m altitude.				

e. Deacclimatization. When altitude-acclimatized personnel descend to low altitude, deacclimatization begins. The rate of deacclimatization is not well known. In well-acclimatized personnel (for example, residents for 16 days at 4,050 m), approximately 50 percent of their altitude acclimatization (that is, absence of AMS and increased SaO_2) was still present after 7 days residing near sea level upon re-ascent to 4,300 m. Altitude acclimatization to moderate altitudes may be lost faster than acclimatization to higher altitudes. The rate of altitude deacclimatization following IHE protocols is not well known, but may be very rapid (that is, 2 to 3 days). It is possible that occasional exposures to high altitude will decrease the rate of deacclimatization, thus extending the duration of effective acclimatization in Soldiers based at low altitudes. Since altitude acclimatization status is not readily measureable at low altitudes, the only notable feature of deacclimatization is an increase in body weight as the plasma volume expands back to normal.

3–3. Monitoring and assessing altitude acclimatization

a. Leaders are responsible for implementing controls to minimize identified risks and for continuously monitoring and evaluating their effectiveness. An important aspect of this implementation is being vigilant for signs of Soldier distress in the altitude environment so that management procedures and interventions can be adjusted accordingly to reduce work impairments and susceptibility to altitude illness. Therefore, all members of a unit must have knowledge of valid metrics for monitoring unit and individual acclimatization status.

b. Written documentation of daily altitude exposure is the best and, at present, the only way to track unit acclimatization status. If units are deployed to terrestrial altitudes above 1,200 m or are passengers on aircraft with cabin altitudes greater than 1,200 m, then a log of their altitude exposure duration can be used to assess their altitude acclimatization status using the information provided in figure 3–1.

c. Currently, there are no tests administered at low altitude that reliably assess a Soldier's altitude acclimatization status. The most objective and quantifiable assessment of altitude acclimatization is ventilatory acclimatization. However, in order to assess ventilatory acclimatization, the Soldier must be exposed to high altitude (real or simulated) during the measurement.

(1) A useful and practical measure of ventilatory acclimatization is resting SaO_2 by pulse oximetry. However, any measurement of SaO_2 by pulse oximetry must be carefully conducted to eliminate possible aberrant results due to cold hands, physical movement artifact, talking, stimulation, voluntary hyperventilation, recent ingestion of food, caffeinated beverages, or recent exercise. A finger pulse oximeter placed on a cold finger will generally underreport the true SaO_2, while all other conditions will elevate the SaO_2 above its true resting value.

(2) A good time to assess resting SaO_2 is immediately upon awakening while the Soldier is still lying in his or her bed or sleeping bag. Table 3–4 lists the expected median resting SaO_2 for unacclimatized and acclimatized individuals over a wide range of altitudes. Soldiers with resting SaO_2 at or below the median value are at greater risk of developing altitude illness than individuals with resting SaO_2 higher than the median SaO_2 for that altitude. Regardless of initial

resting SaO$_2$, each Soldier's SaO$_2$ should increase over 2 to 7 days at a given altitude. Soldiers showing no increase or a decrease in resting SaO$_2$ should be monitored closely for symptoms of altitude illness or other ailments.

   d. At altitudes >3,000 m, resting heart rate is usually elevated during acute exposure and returns to sea-level values with acclimatization. The increase in resting heart rate is proportional to the altitude and ranges from 10 to 30 percent over the Soldier's low-altitude resting heart rate. Because sea-level resting heart rate can vary greatly among Soldiers, trending resting heart rate during altitude exposure must begin at low altitude. The conditions under which resting heart rate is measured must be well controlled and standardized to obtain valid useful data (for example, lying down, immediately upon waking, etc.). Daily measurement and recording of resting heart rate may provide objective evaluation of acclimatization status.

   e. The presence or absence of hypoxic symptoms (lightheadedness, dizziness, fatigue) or altitude illness (for example, AMS) is a useful measure of altitude acclimatization status. Generally, hypoxic and AMS symptoms decline as altitude acclimatization develops. When possible, even during short missions to high altitudes, post-mission debriefings can be used to assess whether an individual experienced any symptoms of hypoxia or AMS.

Table 3–4
Median resting arterial oxyhemoglobin saturation (SaO$_2$) values for unacclimatized and acclimatized personnel at altitude[a]

Value	Personnel	Altitude (m)					
		1,950	2,450	3,050	3,650	4,050	4,500
SaO$_2$ (%)[b]	Unacclimatized	94 (93–95)[b]	94 (93–95)[b]	91 (90–92)[b]	87 (85–89)[b]	82 (80–84)[b]	77 (73–81)[b]
	Acclimatized	94 (93–95)[b]	94 (93–95)[b]	92 (91–93)[b]	89 (88–90)[b]	87 (86–88)[b]	81 (79–83)[b]

Notes:
[a]Soldiers with resting SaO$_2$ values at or below the median value may be at greater risk for developing altitude illness.
[b]In parentheses are 95% confidence levels.

3–4. Pharmaceutical control for altitude stress
Pharmaceutical enhancement of altitude acclimatization is extremely limited. Acetazolamide (Diamox®) is the only medication that induces physiological adaptations similar to altitude acclimatization. For hastening ventilatory acclimatization, acetazolamide administration (250 to 500 milligrams (mg), twice daily (*bis in die* or b.i.d.)) should start at least 24 hrs prior to ascent. Depending upon acetazolamide dosage and target altitude, pharmaceutically aided ventilatory acclimatization is roughly equivalent to 2 to 4 days of continuous altitude residence. After 1 to 2 days at altitude, acetazolamide use can be stopped if symptoms of altitude illness are absent (chapter 6). (Diamox® is a registered trademark of American Cyanamid Company, New York, New York.)

3–5. Supportive interventions

   a. In addition to the procedures described for inducing altitude acclimatization, maintaining adequate hydration levels and primarily consuming carbohydrates can sustain physical performance and possibly decrease altitude illness susceptibility.

   (1) Dehydration significantly impairs physical performance and will increase susceptibility to AMS. The physical performance decrements produced by dehydration are most likely additive to the impairments produced by hypoxia. Dehydration does increase the severity of hypoxic symptoms, such as lightheadedness and dizziness. However, there is no evidence that sustaining a high water intake reduces risk of developing altitude illness. For the same atmospheric climatic conditions (temperature, humidity) and metabolic activity, water requirements may be slightly increased at altitude due to the increased loss of water through breathing and the diuresis produced by hypoxia and/or acetazolamide use. Daily water requirement guidance provided in Technical Bulletin, Medical (TB MED) 507/Air Force Pamphlet (AFPAM) 48–152(I) should be followed with a bias toward the upper range of estimated daily water required as altitude increases.

   (2) Carbohydrate is the most efficient fuel for optimizing physical performance at altitude. A 6-to-12 percent glucose or maltodextran solution in liquid form (for example, 56 grams (g) in 560 millimeters (mm) of water) ingested just before and periodically during moderate to intense physical activity improves endurance performance by 10-to-25 percent at 4,300 m in unacclimatized individuals. Carbohydrate supplementation also maintains blood glucose levels and reduces perception of effort. Moreover, its ingestion after activity completion hastens recovery and replenishment of muscle glycogen stores. In addition to providing energy to power prolonged and intense activity, ingesting carbohydrate in a liquid form assures a better hydration status by replacing much of the fluid volume lost due to sweating and increased ventilation.

   b. Exposure to altitude (continuous or intermittent) stimulates the body to produce more RBCs. This increased erythropoiesis draws on the body's iron stores, potentially causing iron deficiency. Individuals exposed to altitude should maintain an iron-rich diet and/or consider taking an iron supplement.

3–6. Long-term high altitude residence

   a. There have been relatively few prolonged (>month) deployments of U.S. forces to altitudes above 3,000 m. Since the majority of adaptive responses develop within the first weeks of high altitude exposure, a normal healthy Soldier will experience only modest improvements in health or performance with more prolonged residence at high altitudes. Below 5,000 m there are no significant negative consequences of residing at high altitudes for months to a year or more.

   b. Body weight loss is the most commonly observed change with prolonged residence at high to very high altitudes. Chronic mountain sickness has only been observed in life-long residents of high altitudes. Some physical deconditioning will occur at high altitudes since exercise training intensity is reduced (chapter 4). Soldiers will likely require longer times to complete the Army Physical Fitness Test (APFT) 2-mile run at and above 1,400 m.

CHAPTER 4

PHYSICAL PERFORMANCE CAPABILITIES AT ALTITUDE

4–1. General

a. Tactical operations dictate the timing and duration of deployments to mountainous regions. Military personnel will therefore be subjected to hypoxic conditions to which they may not be acclimatized.

b. Hypoxia will immediately impair maximal and prolonged whole-body physical performance capabilities in all personnel by amounts generally proportional to the elevation. Impairments will occur for nearly all tasks but will be most conspicuous for those in which a given distance must be traversed in the shortest time or those that involve sustained or intermittent bouts of arduous physical activities for prolonged durations.

c. The physical performance impairment for a particular task will be variable from one Soldier to another for any elevation above approximately 1,000 m. Specific physiological responses relate to factors such as fitness level, intensity of effort, size of the engaged muscle mass, whether the task requires sustained effort or repeated work/rest cycles, pack load being carried, and amount of acclimatization.

d. The physical performance impairments due solely to hypoxia will be in addition to those associated with terrestrial, logistical, nutritional or altitude illness factors that independently or collectively affect task performance adversely.

e. Task performance will be most impaired in the first few days after rapid deployment from sea level to altitude. Newly arrived military personnel will have difficulty participating in physically demanding tasks or duties such as dismounted patrolling operations, entrenchment, and combat.

f. Maximal physical performance at high altitude is not improved by acclimatization, but may be improved by long-duration (months) residence at moderate altitude.

g. Prolonged physical performance at a given altitude is improved by acclimatization but will remain impaired relative to sea level at elevations above 1,000 m.

h. Hypoxia will minimally impair small muscle mass activity or whole-body activity lasting less than 2 minutes (min).

4–2. Maximal physical performance

a. The O_2 requirement of numerous tasks requiring prolonged, sustained or intermittent activity is often characterized relative to maximal physical performance capability (expressed as VO_{2max} (maximal oxygen uptake)) which is commonly evaluated in an exercise laboratory or can be estimated using a maximal effort 2-mile run (appendix C). Relative intensity (along with heart rate) can then be used at sea level or altitude as general guidance for an individual or unit to estimate task duration or whether assigned tasks should be performed continuously at low intensity or intermittently at a higher intensity alternated with periodic rest periods.

b. When expressed as a unit of body weight (that is, milliliter (mL) of O_2 per kilogram (kg) of body weight per minute or mL/kg/min), VO_{2max} can be used as an index to categorize Soldiers according to their "aerobic fitness" which provides an estimate of their capacity for prolonged work performance. That is, a Soldier with a high VO_{2max} generally can perform a given task that requires a fixed amount of O_2 for a longer period of time than a Soldier with a lower VO_{2max} (that is, the former compared to the latter will be working at a lower percent VO_{2max} and heart rate).

c. At sea level, VO_{2max} is usually—

(1) Higher for men than for women.

(2) Decreased by approximately 9 percent each decade after the age of 25 years.

(3) Increased with regular and intense participation in whole-body, prolonged physical activities such as running or cycling.

(4) Decreased with inactivity.

d. For each Soldier, VO_{2max} represents the functional limit of their respiratory and circulatory systems to deliver O_2 to active muscles and the ability of their active muscles to utilize the O_2 delivered. With increasing elevation, there is a progressive reduction in PB, with resultant declines in inspired, alveolar, and arterial PO_2. As a consequence, VO_{2max} declines for all individuals from sea level at a rate proportional to the increase in altitude. The decline in VO_{2max} at altitude has a direct influence on nearly all tasks performed at altitude.

e. The magnitude of the initial decline in VO_{2max} at a given altitude will not vary with exposure time unless there is a significant change in the frequency, duration, or intensity of athletic training or large reduction in lean body weight due to factors such as inadequate nutrition.

f. Figure 4–1 illustrates that reductions in VO_{2max} are measurable at elevations as low or lower than 580 m, curvilinearly related to elevation, and nearly 80 percent reduced from sea level at the highest elevation on earth (Mount Everest, 8,848 m). Acclimatization has little effect on the relationship between altitude and amount of VO_{2max} decline. Figure 4–1 indicates also that there is a wide variation in VO_{2max} decline at nearly all elevations, especially between 2,000 m and 5,500 m.

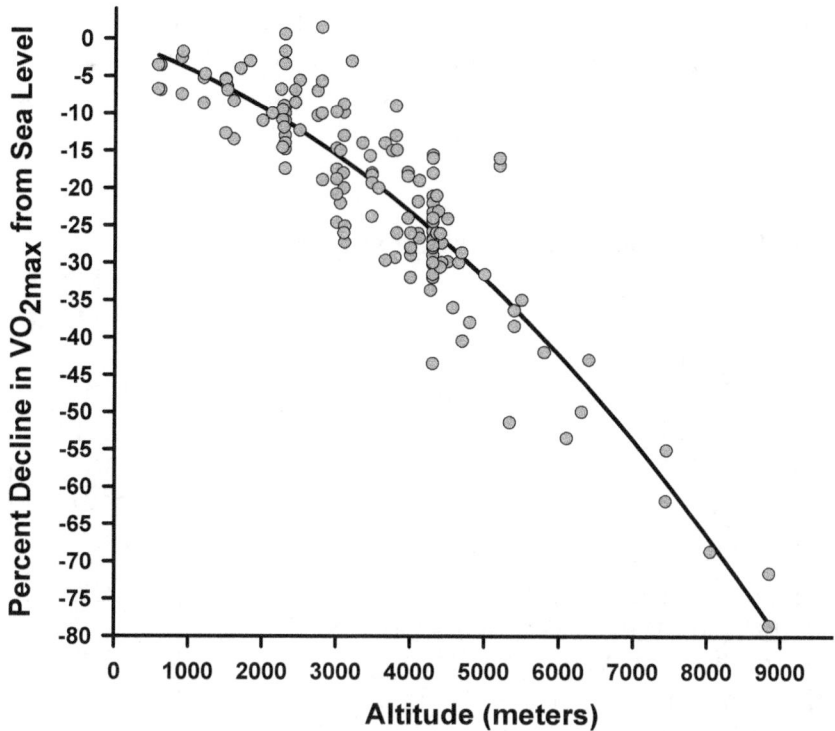

Figure 4–1. Relationship between increasing elevation and decline in maximal oxygen uptake

4-3. Relationship of task performance to maximal oxygen uptake

a. Oxygen is required to perform nearly every physical task with the specific amount ranging from very small (for example, map reading) to extremely large (for example, brisk foot march up a hill with a heavy pack load). If the O_2 requirement of the task is compared to VO_{2max}, the relative intensity (that is, percent VO_{2max}) and the expected heart rate response during performance of the task can be estimated. This information can then be used as general guidance to estimate task duration. For example, a whole-body repetitive task requiring 30 to 40 percent of VO_{2max} (and heart rates of ~100 to 120 beats/min) is a reasonable average upper limit that can be sustained by 20- to 30-year olds over an 8-hr workday for continuous days at sea level. In contrast, whole-body tasks that require more than approximately 40 to 45 percent of VO_{2max} are better suited for shorter durations or for repeated work/rest cycles if they are to be performed over a long period of time.

b. Table 4–1 provides measured percent VO_{2max} values for young Soldiers performing a variety of standardized military tasks that are easy, moderate, and hard for no more than 15 min at sea level. Descriptors such as weight lifted, distance traveled, and activity pace are also provided. The tasks are listed in ascending order of percent VO_{2max}. Note that for any given task, there is a range of percent VO_{2max} values that relate to factors such as VO_{2max}, body size, strength, and gender. Also note that percent VO_{2max} required can differ significantly with seemingly small changes in frequency of lifting (tasks 2 and 5); frequency of lifting and carrying (tasks 3 and 4); weight carried (tasks 7, 10, and 12 and tasks 15 and 17); movement speed (tasks 10 and 15 and tasks 12 and 17); or a difference in terrain (tasks 10 and 16).

Table 4–1
Percentage of maximal oxygen uptake for some military tasks at sea level

Task Number	Task Description	Sea Level % VO_{2max}
	Easy Tasks	
1	Standing in a foxhole/guard duty	9–10
2	Lift and lower, 25 kg, 1.32 m, once/4 min	12–14
3	Lift and carry, 25 kg, 15 m, once/2 min	13–18
4	Lift and carry, 25 kg, 15 m, once/min	16–25
5	Lift and lower, 25 kg, 1.32 m, once/min	18–26
6	Lift 22.7 kg, 1.32 m, twice/min	19–26
7	Load carriage, 4 kilometer (km)/hr, load-bearing equipment only	21–26
8	Two-person litter carry, 68.2 kg, 250 m	22–26
9	Lift 25-kg projectiles, on to a 2.2-ton truck, 1.32 m, twice /min	23–31
10	Load carriage, 4 km/hr, 20-kg load	24–34
11	Lift and carry, 18.2 kg, 9 m, once/min	25–32
	Moderate Tasks	
12	Load carriage, 4 km/hr, 30-kg load	29–40
13	Employ hand grenades, 3 times/min	33–36
14	Dig defensive position, 0.45 m deep, 0.6 m x 1.8 m on sand	33–37
15	Load carriage, 5.3 km/hr, 20-kg load	33–43
16	Load carriage, 1.11 m/seconds, 20-kg load, on loose sand	37–57
	Hard Tasks	
17	Load carriage, 5.3 km/hr, 30-kg load	41–58
18	Four-person litter carry, 81.8 kg, 1000 m	47–54
19	Obstacle course	58–66
20	Move under direct fire (rush/crawl)	59–66

c. Figure 4–2 illustrates the relationship between intensity of effort expressed as a relative O_2 requirement (percent VO_{2max}) for foot marches with load carriage and time to reach exhaustion. The solid line represents the amount of time that a foot march can be performed at various values for percent VO_{2max} before exhaustion occurs. It is important to emphasize that it is the change in intensity by itself rather than the reasons for the change in intensity that ultimately affects time to exhaustion. An increase in either pace or pack load during a foot march will independently increase the intensity of effort as illustrated by percent VO_{2max}. Thus, as pace or load increase, the other has to decrease to maintain the same intensity, the implication being that the total distance traveled over a set period of time also will be changed. For example, the total distance that can be traveled in 6 hrs on level ground without reaching exhaustion will be reduced by ~2 kilometers (km) for every 4.5-km increase in pack weight over 18 kg. Other factors, such as local muscle fatigue and soreness in the legs, hips, lower back and shoulders, loss of agility with increasing loads, blisters, and carrying loads that are awkward or handheld, will independently degrade performance.

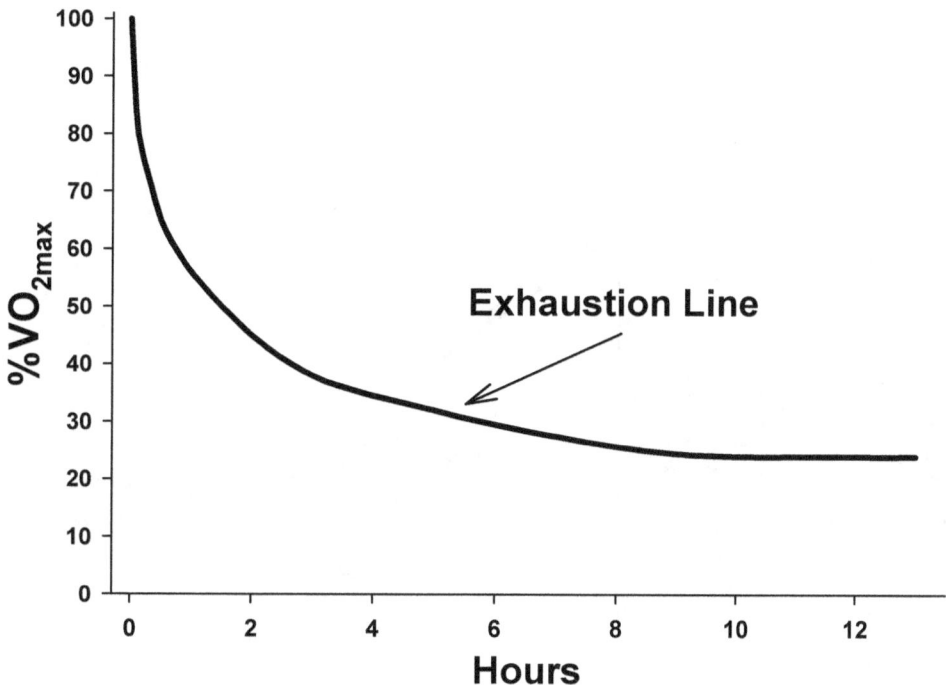

Figure 4–2. Relationship between intensity of pack load carriage effort (percent maximal oxygen uptake) and time to reach exhaustion

4–4. Effect of altitude on prolonged physical performance

a. The decline in VO_{2max} at altitude directly affects performance of nearly all tasks. The O_2 requirement for any given prolonged task that is performed at a specified rate or pace is similar at sea level and altitude. But because VO_{2max} progressively decreases with increasing elevation, the O_2 requirement of the task will represent a relatively greater percent VO_{2max} with increasing elevation.

b. Figure 4–3 illustrates the consequences of a Soldier performing a prolonged task (for example, load carriage) at sea level and during initial exposure to 4,300 m altitude. In both locations, the O_2 requirement to perform the task is identical at 2 liters per minute (L/min), but VO_{2max} is reduced from sea level to altitude by 27 percent (4.2 L/min to 3.1 L/min). Thus, the percent VO_{2max} or relative intensity has been significantly increased from 50 percent at sea level to 68 percent at altitude and will therefore be perceived as far more difficult to perform at the same rate. In addition, various physiological indices associated with a higher percent VO_{2max}, such as muscle glycogen utilization, blood lactate, ventilation, and heart rate, will also be higher compared to sea level.

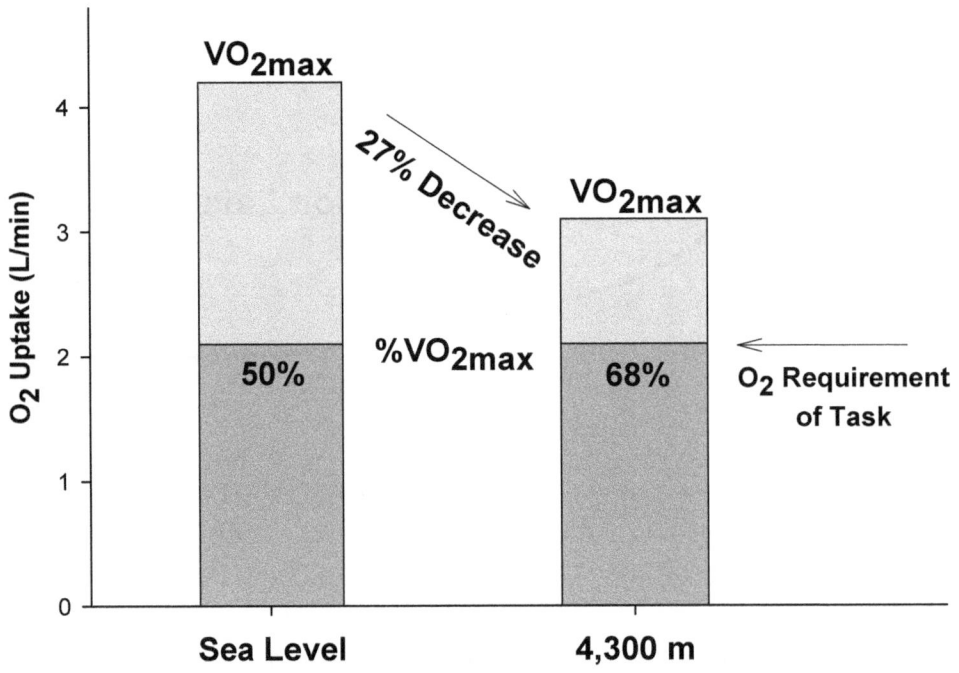

Figure 4–3. Increase in percent maximal oxygen uptake despite no change in task requirement at 4,300 meters

c. Most tasks become progressively more difficult with increasing elevation. Many military operations are performed by a unit, with each Soldier within the unit performing a single or series of tasks. As such, the interaction of differing individual increases in relative intensity with an increase in elevation can introduce significant limitations for the timely and planned completion of the entire operation. When Soldiers with a high VO_{2max} work together with Soldiers with a low VO_{2max}, a hard task that might be sustainable for an hour or so at sea level will not be sustained for more than a couple of minutes at very high altitudes.

d. Figure 4–4 shows that with each subsequent 1,000-m increase in elevation from sea level, the amount of time that the collective pace of the operation can be maintained at a maximal-effort, sea-level tempo is reduced progressively with increasing elevation.

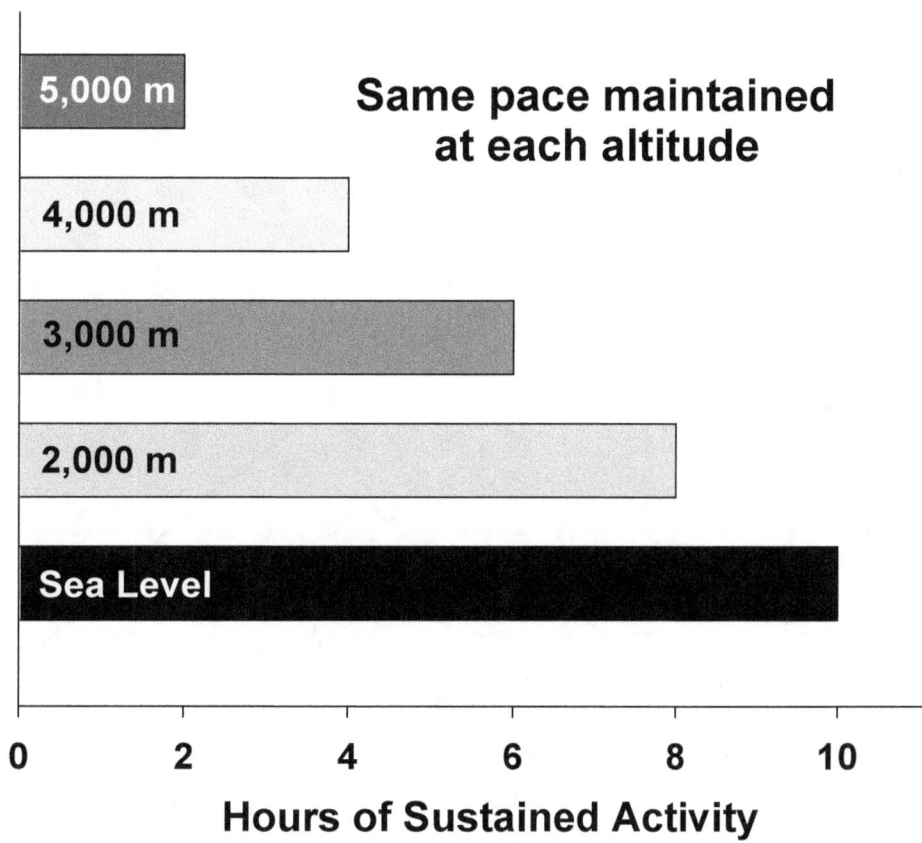

Figure 4–4. The effect of increasing elevation on sustained task duration

e. It is clear that an increase in elevation increases percent VO_{2max} and reduces the amount of time that a task can be performed at the same pace as at sea level. Therefore, to successfully complete the tasks, at least one of the following time-based modifications must be included in operational planning at altitude: reduce task intensity or pace, or allow more frequent or longer rest breaks. Any or all of these modifications will increase the time to complete most tasks during any mountain operation. Thus, the number of planned daily tasks performed by a Soldier or unit at altitude will have to be reduced from the number that can be performed at sea level.

f. Figure 4–5 shows how foot march pace is reduced with increasing elevation even after acclimatization. Values for percent VO_{2max} and heart rate were assumed to be maintained similarly at each elevation during the ascent as they were at sea level. Figure 4–5 represents only the performance impairment due to hypoxia. Other factors such as altitude illness, grade of ascent, environmental and trail conditions, inadequate nutrition, technical difficulty, lack of acclimatization, or additional clothing and equipment would reduce the foot march pace even more.

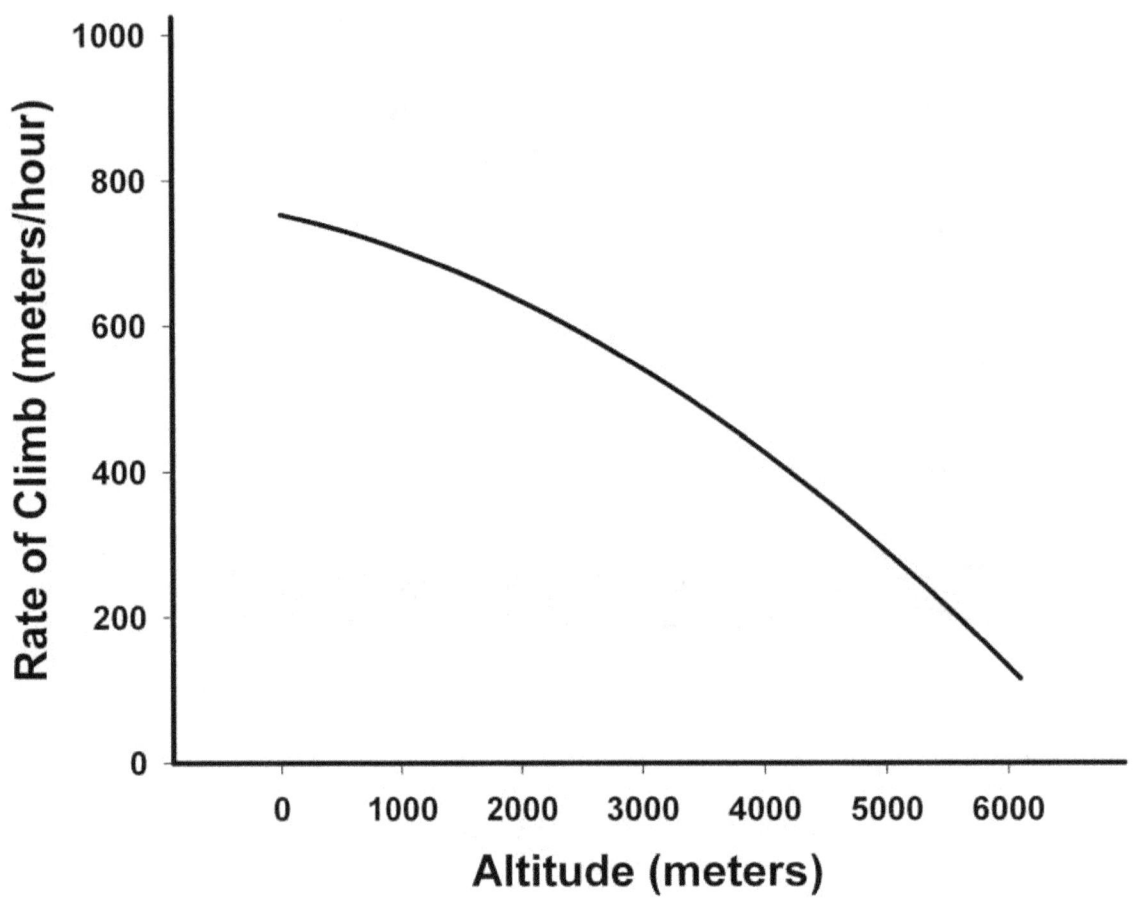

Figure 4–5. Reduction in climbing rate with increasing elevation due to hypoxia in acclimatized Soldiers

g. It is important to emphasize that while the absolute amount of work will necessarily be reduced at altitude compared to sea level, the relative relationship among percent VO_{2max}, heart rate, and perception of difficulty will be similar at sea level and during early altitude exposure; thus, at least one value will provide an estimate of the others. This relationship will change with acclimatization, however. That is, heart rate and perception of difficulty will be reduced after acclimatization if the task is performed at the same percent VO_{2max} as during early exposure. The implication is that if values for heart rate and/or perception of difficulty are similarly maintained throughout the altitude exposure, Soldiers will be performing the task at an acceptably higher percent VO_{2max} after acclimatization than they did during earlier exposure. Thus, heart rate monitoring provides a means to assure that the task is being performed at a pace that is appropriate and acceptable for the current level of acclimatization.

h. The specific amount and type of time modification to the operational planning of various tasks at altitude will depend on factors such as range of physical capabilities of the deployed unit, task difficulty, elevation, acclimatization, experience, urgency, weather, terrain, size of involved muscle mass, and load carried. Because of these factors, precise time adjustments for particular tasks for specific altitudes and how these adjustments may affect unit operation effectiveness are difficult to predict prior to deployment. Nevertheless, additional time to complete various tasks with initial exposure and after significant acclimatization at the same altitudes can be estimated. Table 4–2 summarizes the estimated percentage time increases at altitudes ranging from 1,000 m to 5,000 m for whole-body tasks having durations at sea level of <2 min, 2 to 5 min, 20 to 30 min, and >2 hrs. Values are provided for initial exposure and after 10 days of acclimatization resulting from living at the same elevation. In general—

(1) Tasks that are less than 2 min in duration are little affected at any of the altitudes listed.

(2) For tasks lasting 2 min or longer, the time to complete the tasks increases progressively with elevation.

(3) The longer the task duration, the greater the percentage increase in time to complete the task at any elevation compared to sea level, even after acclimatization.

(4) Acclimatization at each elevation reduces the amount of time required to complete all tasks greater than 2 min. With increasing elevation, the improvement (that is, percentage reduction in task duration) becomes progressively greater with acclimatization.

Table 4–2
Estimated percent increases in times to complete tasks of differing durations relative to sea level

Altitude (m)	Percentage Increases in Task Durations for Unacclimatized and Acclimatized Individuals							
	<2 min		2–5 min		20–30 min		>2 hrs	
	Initial	>10 d	Initial	>10 d	Initial	>10 d	Initial	>10 d
1,000	0	0	2	0	4	1	5	2
2,000	0	0	7	2	11	4	18	12
3,000	0	0	12	5	20	12	40	28
4,000	2	0	18	9	45	20	65	45
5,000	2	0	50	25	90	60	200	90

Legend:
d=days

4–5. Time estimation of a unit foot march on mountain trails

a. Historically, map distance plus one-third of the map distance has been used as a general guide to estimate actual ground distance to be traveled on dirt trails through the mountains. The added distance accounts for minor ascents and descents and non-linearity of routes inherent to mountainous terrain.

b. In addition, 1 hr is commonly added to the time required to cover the ground distance for each 300 m of ascent or 600 m of descent.

c. With increasing elevations, additional time should also be added to account for the likely hypoxia-induced reduction in pace and increased number or duration of rest periods during travel on flat and ascending terrain. No hypoxia adjustment is needed for the descent.

d. A slow, steady pace is preferred to more rapid movement with frequent stops. Also, the collective pace will be slower as the unit increases in size. A typical pace for an 8- to 12-person squad carrying a light load is 4 km/hr including 5 to 10 min of rest for every ½ hr of foot march. Following is an example using Soldiers having high VO_{2max} values.

(1) Information provided. The map distance is 12 km. There are 600 m of ascent and 600 m of descent, with an average elevation of 3,000 m. Average foot march pace for the squad is 4 km/hr over a dirt trail carrying a pack weighing 22 km that requires 28 percent of VO_{2max} on level ground and 50 percent of VO_{2max} while ascending. (Note: The example provided here is for foot marching only. More advanced mountaineering tasks such as rock climbing, belaying and rappelling required in some mountain environments will add more time to the estimate as a direct result of performing the task and also indirectly because of the heavier load carried due to the additional weight of technical equipment.)

(2) Calculations. Ground distance is estimated as 16 km (map distance plus one-third of map distance). The 600-m ascent requires an additional 2 hrs (600 m/300 m per hr), and the 600-m descent requires an additional hour (600 m/600 m per hr). The final estimated duration to complete the ground distance and the ascent has been increased by 28 percent and 40 percent for acclimatized and unacclimatized Soldiers, respectively (see table 4–2). The estimated overall duration will therefore be approximately 1.7 and 2.4 hrs (or 24 and 34 percent) longer, respectively, at 3,000 m than for elevations less than 1,000 m over similar terrain. The calculations are summarized in table 4–3. Time estimates for the unit foot march should be modified if factors, such as elevation, pack load, grade, unit fitness, number of participants, pace or trail surface, differ from those provided in the above example.

Table 4–3
Estimated time to complete a 16-kilometer foot march near sea level and 3,000 meters

	Distance	<1,000 m (hrs)	3,000 m Acclimatized (hrs)	3,000 m Unacclimatized (hrs)
Ground Distance	16 km	4.0	5.1	5.6
Ascent	600 m	2.0	2.6	2.8
Descent	600 m	1.0	1.0	1.0
Totals		**7.0**	**8.7**	**9.4**

4–6. Physical performance, weight loss, nutrition, and acetazolamide

a. Soldiers deployed to high mountainous areas are likely to be in negative energy balance for weeks or longer and will lose body weight. The energy deficit is usually attributed to some combination of voluntarily or involuntarily reduced consumption of field rations, altitude illness, diuresis, increased time being physically active, heavier loads being carried, and elevation of basal metabolic rate. Body weight losses of approximately 5 percent or less are typical and usually do not affect performance of most tasks.

b. There is little indication that altitude exposure by itself requires supplementation of protein, vitamins or minerals (other than iron).

c. A negative energy balance is usually also associated with reduced carbohydrate intakes that are much less than the recommended minimum of 400 g per day. A consistently diminished daily carbohydrate intake results in reduced muscle glycogen storage that will likely contribute to diminished performance especially during prolonged, difficult tasks. A carbohydrate-rich diet, as well as frequent ingestion of small amounts of carbohydrate-rich foods or liquids during prolonged, difficult tasks, will sustain performance at the highest level possible for a given altitude.

d. Caffeine ingested prior to participating in some prolonged tasks at altitude may help sustain performance. However, for some Soldiers, there will be increased diuresis that may exacerbate an already present altitude-induced hypohydration. Therefore, caffeine should be consumed in moderation at altitude.

e. There is no evidence that creatine supplementation will improve task performance at altitude.

f. Acetazolamide is often provided for the avoidance/treatment of altitude illness during early exposure to altitude (see chapter 6). However, acetazolamide will worsen performance of high intensity tasks that involve either prolonged whole-body effort or rapidly repeated local muscular effort. Moreover, paresthesia (that is, tingling) in the extremities that occurs during acetazolamide treatment typically becomes more pronounced with increased effort and may be bothersome during tasks requiring fine motor control.

4–7. Physical training while deployed at altitude

  a. Endurance training.

  (1) Monitoring heart rate provides a safe, easy and objective means to maintain the proper exercise intensity during endurance training while deployed at altitudes up to approximately 4,000 m, as it does at sea level. That is, approximately the same heart rate range, duration, and frequency that was used during training at sea level can be used up to 4,000 m. For example, a commonly used formula of (220 – age) times 55 percent and 90 percent estimates that training heart rate for ~ 20-year-olds should be maintained in the range of 110 to 180 beats per min for 20 to 60 min per day for 3 or more days per week. Doing so will provide the necessary training stimulus to at least maintain endurance fitness. For the same perceived effort, jogging pace will be reduced at altitude compared to sea level.

  (2) For the first few days of rapid exposure to moderate to high elevations, all voluntary activity should be minimized and endurance training stopped or intensity greatly reduced to minimize susceptibility to altitude illness.

  (3) After the first few days, endurance training can resume. For the first couple of sessions, training heart rate should be maintained in the lower part of the heart rate range, with the training session duration being no more than approximately 30 minutes. As altitude acclimatization develops, heart rate and the duration and frequency of the exercise sessions can be progressively increased as desired.

  b. Strength training.

  (1) For the first few days of rapid exposure to moderate to high elevations, all voluntary activity should be minimized and strength training stopped to reduce susceptibility to altitude illness.

  (2) After this time, strength training can resume as at sea level. It is not necessary to monitor heart rate during strength training. The amount of weight, sets, and repetitions used during each exercise session should be similar at altitude and at sea level. Required rest periods between sets likely will be slightly longer.

  c. Stretch training. Muscle stretching exercise (for example, yoga) can be performed without restriction.

CHAPTER 5

NEUROPSYCHOLOGICAL PERFORMANCE AT ALTITUDE

5–1. General

a. Altitude stress can cause a wide range of neuropsychological consequences that affect a Soldier's mood, senses, judgment, memory and ability to perform cognitive and psychomotor tasks. Generally, significant changes in neuropsychological function emerge at altitudes higher than 3,000 m. However, Soldiers who have low levels of ventilation or impaired pulmonary gas exchange may experience neuropsychological problems at even lower altitudes. Changes in neuropsychological function are most evident in unacclimatized Soldiers during the first 24 hrs of their ascent above 3,000 m. Also, there is a progression in the deleterious effects of hypoxia on the central nervous system. The higher cortical centers are the most sensitive, followed by the cerebellum, medulla, and spinal cord. Higher-level brain functions involving cognition, decision-making, and reasoning are most sensitive to the effects of altitude and oxygen deprivation. Figure 5–1 indicates the general progression in deterioration of sensory and mental function with increasing hypoxia. Reductions are presented relative to sea-level function in figure 5–1.

b. Sleep deprivation, poor sleep quality and quantity, and physical fatigue will contribute to the direct effects of hypoxia on neuropsychological function. Sleep quality and quantity are decreased at altitude due to increased awakenings resulting from central sleep apnea. Soldiers experiencing more frequent awakenings demonstrate greater impairments in cognition. Hypoventilation during sleep increases the severity of hypoxemia. Increased hypoxemia can contribute directly to increased neuropsychological impairments as well as increased AMS severity (chapter 6). Hypoxia increases the development and feeling of physical fatigue both by direct effects on the brain and by lowering the maximal oxygen uptake of the warfighter at altitude (chapter 4). Fatigue also contributes to decreased motivation that can adversely impact cognitive and psychomotor performances at altitude.

5–2. Mood states and personality

a. Changes in mood states and personality are usually not recognized by the affected Soldier. Initially, Soldiers can exhibit euphoria that can lead to overconfidence. After several hours at altitude, Soldiers may become irritable, quarrelsome, uncooperative, anxious, apathetic, and less friendly and clear thinking. More adverse changes are noted at altitudes above 4,000 m. These aversive mood changes reach a peak after 18 to 24 hrs of altitude exposure and recede to normal after 48 hrs, at altitudes up to 4,700 m. Moods of Soldiers afflicted with severe AMS are more negative and improve more slowly than individuals with no illness. These behaviors are usually not acknowledged by the affected Soldiers and may even be adamantly denied. Unit leaders must anticipate these mood changes and their potential impact on unit cohesion. Altitude acclimatization lessens these adverse changes in mood states. Acetazolamide (used to prevent AMS) will lessen the intensity of these adverse mood changes (chapter 6).

b. Changes in personality are minimal below 5,000 m. At and above this altitude, personality changes may include paranoia, obsessive-compulsiveness, depression, hostility, eroded self-confidence, and nervous exhaustion. After exposure to extreme altitude, Soldiers' self-ratings of their abilities improve (that is, increased self-esteem), but their acceptance of others in the altitude expedition decreases. While these changes in personality may have resulted from high altitude by itself, the heavy physical demands, enforced intragroup dependence, close living quarters, cold temperatures, sensory deprivation, and frequent periods of reduced visual fields may also contribute.

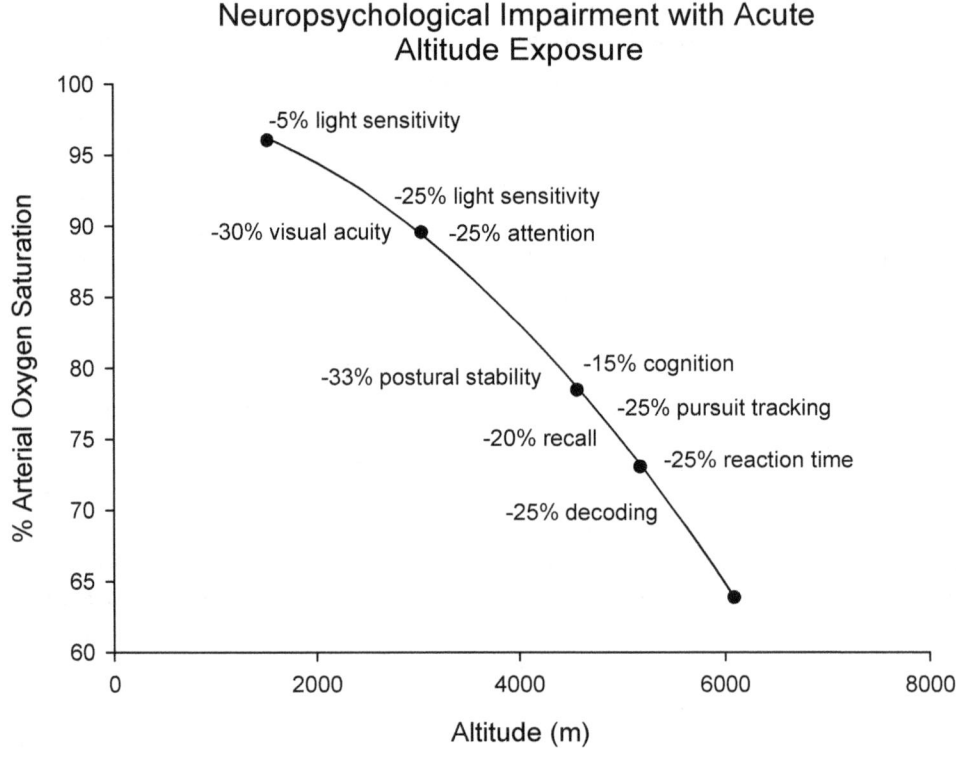

Figure 5–1. Effect of increasing altitude on several sensory and neurocognitive functions

5–3. Special senses

a. Of the special senses (vision, hearing, smell, taste, and touch), vision is the most sensitive to the effects of hypoxia. Decrements in light sensitivity can occur at altitudes as low as 1,525 m (figure 5–1). Visual acuity and color discrimination are measurably decreased above 3,000 m. Above 4,000 m, the combination of impaired dark adaptation and decreased accommodation and convergence lead to increased occurrence of heterophorias. From moderate to extreme altitude, night vision (light sensitivity and visual acuity) is more affected than daytime vision. There appears to be little recovery of visual function with development of altitude acclimatization.

However, visual function rapidly returns to normal with either descent or supplemental oxygen. There are no pharmaceutical or nutritional interventions that will improve visual function at altitude.

b. Visual performance through night vision goggles decreases at altitudes above 3,000 m, although less than unaided night vision.

c. The direct effects of hypoxia on visual function can be exacerbated by the typical lack of common terrain features and the bright sunlight of high mountainous areas. Lack of common terrain features (for example, trees, buildings, etc.) can adversely impair depth perception. Because there is less light scatter and brighter sunlight at altitude, the contrast between the sunlit and shadowed areas increases.

d. These impairments in visual performance at altitude can adversely affect any psychomotor or cognitive tasks (for example, vigilance, eye-hand coordination, target detection, etc.) that involve borderline light conditions, even at moderate altitudes.

e. Systemic hypoxia causes an increase in retinal blood flow. Upon ophthalmic examination, retinal arterioles appear darker (cyanotic) and engorged (swollen). Occasionally, small hemorrhages will be observed (chapter 6).

f. Hearing exhibits little or no decrements until very high altitudes (>4,600 m) are attained.

g. Taste sensation (salty, sour, bitter and sweet) diminishes with increasing altitude. This may contribute to high altitude anorexia (chapter 6).

h. There are no known deficits in the special senses of smell and touch at altitude.

5–4. Cognitive and psychomotor performance

a. Altitudes above 3,000 m can produce substantial impairments in a number of cognitive and psychomotor performance measures. Cognitive performance is more affected at altitude than psychomotor performance, and complex tasks are usually affected before simple tasks. Successful execution of many military tasks is dependent upon the integration of multiple cognitive functions.

b. Cognitive and psychomotor performance changes do not follow the same time course at altitude as do symptoms of AMS. Within minutes of exposure to altitudes above 3,000 m, cognitive and psychomotor performances decrease, whereas development of AMS may not occur for 4 or more hrs. At altitudes below 5,000 m, cognitive performances improve and return toward baseline after 24 to 48 hrs. Cognitive performances improve less in individuals afflicted with AMS during this period. Soldiers afflicted with severe AMS will have greater impairment of cognitive performances than Soldiers with lesser symptoms. Upon return to low altitude, cognitive and psychomotor performances quickly return to normal. However, some cases of long-term to permanent cognitive impairments have been reported in climbers who ascended to extreme altitudes (>5,500 m).

c. Tasks requiring assimilation of novel information and/or requiring decisions and strategies (for example, friend-foe identification, targeting, tactical maneuvering, etc.) are more vulnerable to hypoxia than simple and more automated tasks (for example, weapon function check, donning mission-oriented protective posture gear, etc.). Performances involving visual processing of shapes, patterns, and contours are more affected at altitude than those involving numbers, words or characters. Vigilance is decreased and may be related to the fatigue or lethargy caused by hypoxia. Psychomotor tasks, such as choice reaction time, finger dexterity, and arm-hand coordination, are degraded above 3,000 m but to a lesser extent than cognitive performance tasks. There are no validated predictive models of cognitive and psychomotor performances as a function of altitude and exposure duration. Given the progressive severity of hypoxia with increasing altitude, adverse changes in cognitive and psychomotor performances are expected to be greater at progressively higher altitudes. Sleep deprivation and fragmented sleep caused by hypoxia may also contribute to reduced cognitive and psychomotor performances at high altitudes.

d. Cognitive performance impairments at altitude result from either decreased accuracy (that is, increased errors), slowing of performance (that is, decreased speed), or a combination of both. Most cognitive performance impairments at altitude result primarily from a slowing of performance rather than decreased accuracy. However, more errors are likely to occur at altitude when tasks are paced by external conditions. The goal of the task can also alter the tradeoff between accuracy and speed on task impairment at altitude. For example, during a marksmanship task with a goal of hitting as many targets as possible within a prescribed period, time taken to sight the target was reduced, and accuracy was less than sea-level performance.

5–5. Mitigation of neuropsychological impairments

a. The effects of altitude on mood states, and visual, cognitive and psychomotor performances are often larger than those recognized by the affected Soldier(s). Unit leaders must anticipate these adverse changes and their potential impact on unit effectiveness. Because everyone at altitude is susceptible to these adverse changes, the buddy system may not be as effective in recognizing and controlling the adverse impact of altitude on neuropsychological function. Increased monitoring of individual and unit actions by observers at lower altitudes may help identify neuropsychological impairments. This approach is frequently employed by climbing teams at extreme altitudes where team leaders or physicians at base camp monitor the progress and performance of the climbing team and make decisions to minimize risk to the climbing team.

> **NEUROPSYCHOLOGICAL PERFORMANCE**
> Key Points
> - Decrements emerge at altitudes >3,000 m.
> - *Everyone* is susceptible.
> - Aversive moods are common.
> - Decreased night visual performance.
> - Impaired complex task performance.
> - Reduced vigilance.
> - Worst in Soldiers suffering AMS.
> - Well-learned/practiced procedures less affected by altitude.
> - Minimize by staging, graded ascent, and acetazolamide.

b. For military units, the most practical approaches to minimize adverse effects include acclimatization and psychological and medical strategies.

(1) The most effective strategy to mitigate adverse neuropsychological changes is physiological acclimatization to the operational altitude. Guidance on acclimatization procedures is provided in chapter 3. With specific regard to cognitive and psychomotor performances, beneficial effects occur within 1 to 2 days of residence at altitudes up to about 4,500 m. Beneficial changes in mood states may require 3 or more days of acclimatization. Visual function does not improve with altitude acclimatization.

(2) Psychological strategies use training and familiarization with the adverse effects of the altitude environment, together with greater tolerance of the unpleasant symptoms caused by the hypoxic environment, to develop compensatory practices and behaviors. Failure to perceive the consequences of ill-performed routine tasks taken for granted at sea level could have dire consequences for missions at altitude. Learning and regularly performing tasks well at low altitude helps sustain task performance at altitude. Experience performing tasks at altitude helps to develop coping strategies that mitigate impairments on task performance. Experiencing the symptoms and discomforts of the altitude environment will facilitate subsequent coping in this environment. Risk management controls, such as checklists and standing operating procedures, can be developed to ensure critical procedures are properly performed at altitude.

(3) Medical strategies to prevent neuropsychological impairments at altitude are limited. Supplemental oxygen is the most effective therapeutic at altitude. Caffeine ingestion will improve vigilance. Reduction or prevention of AMS using acetazolamide can help ameliorate adverse moods, but has little direct effect on cognitive or psychomotor performances. Dexamethasone will reduce adverse moods, impairments in cognitive or psychomotor performances, and prevent or treat AMS and high altitude cerebral edema (HACE). This drug must be used with caution (chapter 6).

This page intentionally left blank

CHAPTER 6

HIGH ALTITUDE ILLNESS: IDENTIFICATION AND TREATMENT

6–1. Medical problems in high mountain areas

a. Medical problems (other than ballistic injuries) in Soldiers operating in high mountain environments can be classified into three broad categories—

(1) Problems caused by sustained hypobaric hypoxia.

(2) Problems caused by environmental and mission factors.

(3) Exacerbation of preexisting medical conditions (table 6–1).

b. Problems caused by sustained hypobaric hypoxia are unique to high altitudes, and medical personnel may be unfamiliar with them. Medical personnel are more familiar with environmental injuries (such as sunburn and dehydration) and preexisting medical conditions that can occur in many different environments. Problems not directly caused by hypobaric hypoxia can be profoundly affected by it, and medical personnel must be aware of that potential. Appendix D presents a summary of treatments for some of the problems that are commonly encountered in high mountainous areas.

c. Medical problems related to sustained hypobaric hypoxia are often termed high altitude illnesses (appendix E). They range in incidence from common to rare and in severity from benign to rapidly fatal. The incidence and severity are a function of the magnitude of the hypoxic stress as determined by the altitude, the rate of ascent, and the length of exposure (hours, days, months). Factors that contribute to the severity of symptoms include—

(1) The level of physical exertion.

(2) Individual susceptibility.

(3) Body mass index.

(4) Age.

(5) Coexisting medical problems.

d. The most common high altitude illnesses are AMS, HACE, HAPE, altitude-induced peripheral edema (AIPE), and high altitude retinal hemorrhage (HARH).

e. All high altitude illnesses are related to sustained hypoxia and can be treated by raising O_2 levels to the body tissues. Although this can be accomplished using supplemental O_2, the preferred management for all high altitude illnesses is evacuation to a lower altitude.

Table 6–1
Medical problems in military personnel exposed to high mountain environments

Hypobaric Hypoxia Related	Environmental/Mission Factors	Preexisting Medical Conditions
Acute Mountain Sickness	Trauma	Hematologic Conditions
High Altitude Cerebral Edema	Cold Injury	Respiratory Conditions
High Altitude Pulmonary Edema	Heat Injury	Cardiovascular Conditions
Altitude-Induced Peripheral Edema	Solar Radiation Injury	Neurologic Conditions
High Altitude Retinal Hemorrhage	Lightning Strikes	Metabolic Conditions
High Altitude Pharyngitis/Bronchitis	Carbon Monoxide Poisoning	Eye Conditions
Sleep Disturbances	Infectious Disease	Psychiatric Conditions
Blood-clotting Disorders	Dehydration	Gastrointestinal Conditions
Subacute Mountain Sickness	Negative Energy Balance	Pregnancy
Immune Suppression/Wound Healing	Constipation and Hemorrhoids	Pharmacologically Active Substances

6–2. Hypobaric-hypoxia medical problems

  a. Acute mountain sickness (AMS).

  (1) Acute mountain sickness occurs in Soldiers from low altitude (<1,200 m) who ascend rapidly to high altitude (>2,500 m) or from high to higher altitude and remain there for several hours or more. Acute mountain sickness is caused by the decreased amount of O_2 available to the body in the low-pressure atmosphere at high altitude. The pathophysiology of AMS is thought to be the result of mild cerebral edema and subsequent brain swelling. Although not life-threatening, AMS is the most common altitude illness, and its symptoms, when severe, can degrade physical and mental performance such that large numbers of troops may be completely incapacitated in their first few days at altitude. In a few Soldiers, AMS can progress to life-threatening HACE or HAPE, both of which require evacuation.

(2) The incidence and severity of AMS symptoms vary with the altitude, the rate of ascent, length of exposure, level of physical exertion, recent altitude exposure, and individual susceptibility. The higher the altitude, the higher the incidence and severity of AMS (table 6–2). The faster the ascent (that is, vigorous activity), the higher the incidence and severity of AMS (table 6–3). Recent exposure to altitude provides some protection against AMS. Some Soldiers are more susceptible than others and experience the same symptoms on repeated exposures. There is no way to predict susceptibility except from an individual's previous experience. Older men and women appear to be less susceptible and obese individuals more susceptible. Exposure to cold environmental conditions appears to increase susceptibility. Although an association between AMS and dehydration has been noted, it is unclear whether dehydration is an independent risk factor. Neither a Soldier's level of physical fitness, gender, or menstrual cycle phase appears to influence susceptibility.

Table 6–2
Estimated acute mountain sickness incidence and severity in unacclimatized Soldiers rapidly ascending to altitude from below 1,200 meters

Altitude	Incidence (%)		
	Mild	**Moderate**	**Severe**
2,500–3,000 m	10–30	10–20	0–10
3,000–3,500 m	10–40	20–40	10–20
3,500–4,000 m	10–30	40–60	20–30
4,000–4,500 m	10–20	20–40	30–40
>4,500 m	0	10–20	>70

(3) Signs and symptoms of AMS are listed in table 6–3. Headache is the cardinal symptom of AMS and is usually accompanied by insomnia, unusual fatigue, dizziness, anorexia, and nausea. Acute mountain sickness is not accompanied by abnormal neurological findings such as ataxia or altered mental status. The onset of AMS symptoms occurs 4 to 24 hrs after ascent to high altitude, reaches peak severity in 24 to 48 hrs, and subsides over 3 to 7 days at the same altitude. Further ascent without an acclimatization period usually exacerbates symptoms and can result in increased incidence of HAPE or HACE. The majority of AMS cases do not progress to more serious altitude illness without continued ascent.

Table 6–3
Frequency of symptoms in active mountain trekkers and inactive tourists with acute mountain sickness

Symptom	Frequency (%)	
	Trekkers (Active)	Tourists (Inactive)
Headache	96	62
Insomnia	70	31
Anorexia	38	11
Nausea	35	...
Dizziness	27	21
Dyspnea on exertion	25	21
Reduced urinary output	20	...
Marked lassitude	13	...
Vomiting	14	3
Incoordination	11	...

(4) Diagnosis of AMS is based on the occurrence of headache and at least one other sign or symptom in a setting of recent gain in altitude. The Lake Louise AMS Scoring System (appendix F) consists of a five-question self-reported assessment of AMS symptoms with scores ≥ 3 plus headache diagnostic of AMS. The second part of the questionnaire is useful for identifying the progression of AMS to HACE because mental status and gait ataxia are assessed. An added advantage of the Lake Louise AMS Scoring System is that the score can be easily derived. Moreover, the self-reported portion of the Lake Louise AMS Scoring System allows classification of AMS as mild (Lake Louise Scoring System (LLS) <4), moderate (LLS ≥4 but ≤8), and severe (LLS >8). This classification aids in determining treatment options.

(5) Differential diagnosis of AMS includes viral flu-like illness, alcohol hangover, exhaustion, migraine, hypothermia, CO poisoning, and/or dehydration (figure 6–1). Symptoms suggestive of AMS in a setting of recent gain in altitude are probably AMS and should be treated as such until proven otherwise. All misdiagnoses must be eliminated by a physical exam, history, or treatment. Fever is usually absent in AMS, and alcohol or other drug use can be excluded by history. Rest and rehydration can eliminate fatigue and dehydration in the differential diagnosis. Hypothermia is usually accompanied by a decrease in body temperature. Carbon monoxide poisoning can be excluded by a history of recent exposure in a tent, cave, or vehicle with a heater, stove or a running motor. Onset of symptoms more than 3 days after arrival at high altitude, the absence of headache, a rapid response to fluids or rest, and the absence of a response to descent, supplemental O_2, or hyperbaric chamber therapy all suggest other diagnoses. Gait ataxia and mental confusion are indicative of progression to HACE. Dyspnea at rest and dry cough are indicative of progression to HAPE. See figure 6–1 for an overview of the decision tree for the differential diagnosis of AMS.

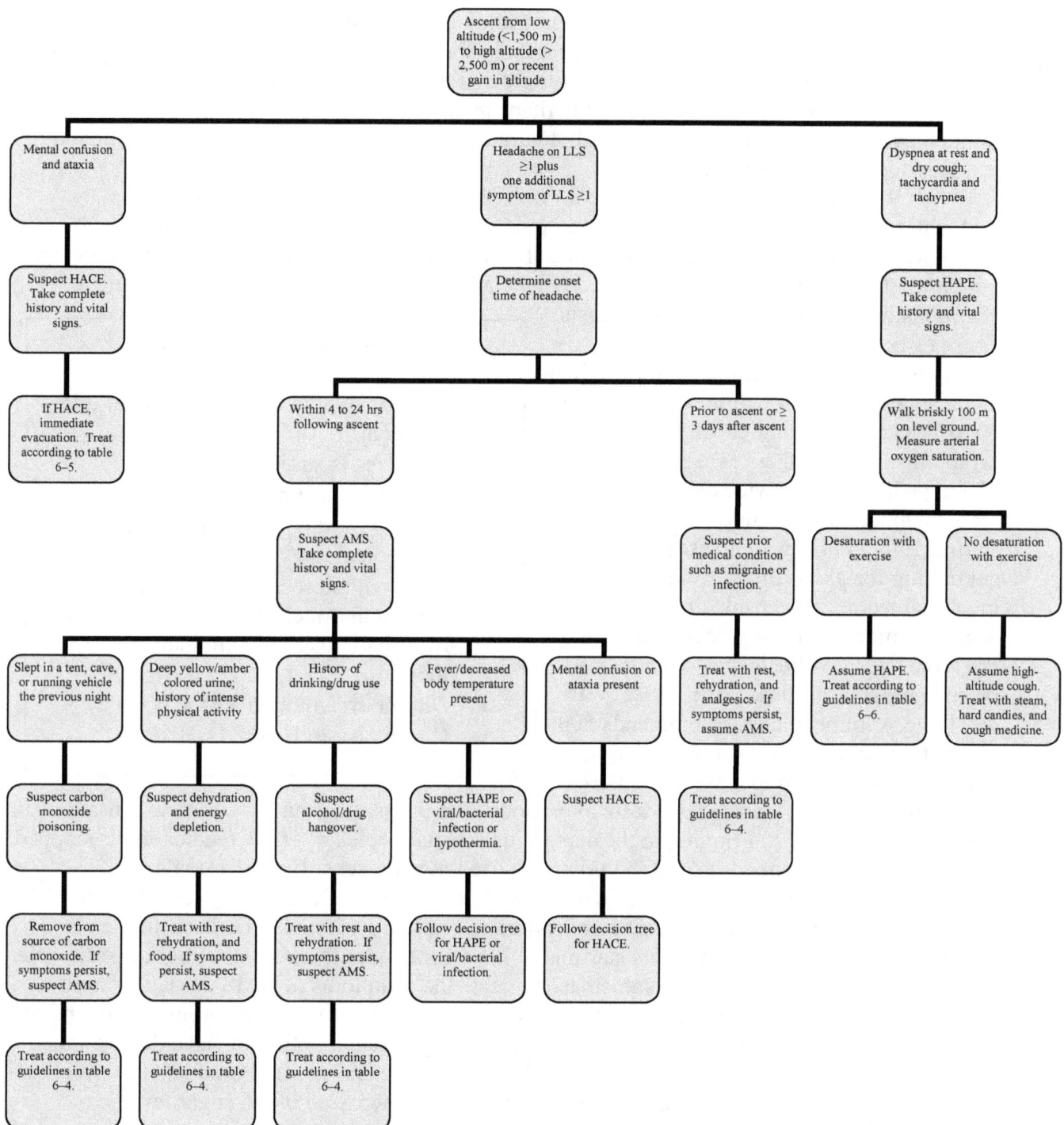

Figure 6–1. Decision tree for differential diagnosis of acute mountain sickness

(6) Prevention of AMS includes non-pharmacologic and pharmacologic methods. Non-pharmacologic methods that promote acclimatization are the safest and most effective means for preventing AMS, but they take time to accomplish, and sufficient time may not be available in many operational scenarios. Non-pharmacologic methods to prevent AMS include staged and graded ascent, avoiding overexertion and perhaps intermittent hypoxic exposure (see chapter 3). Limited evidence suggests that a high carbohydrate diet is another non-pharmacologic method that may reduce symptoms of AMS.

(a) When there is insufficient time for non-pharmacologic methods to induce acclimatization, Soldiers may use pharmacologic prophylaxis to prevent AMS. The drug of choice for preventing AMS is acetazolamide (Diamox®). Acetazolamide is a carbonic anhydrase inhibitor and reduces reabsorption of bicarbonate and sodium in the kidney, thus causing a bicarbonate diuresis and metabolic acidosis. These effects rapidly enhance both ventilatory and renal acclimatization. When taken appropriately, it will prevent AMS in 50 to 75 percent of Soldiers and reduce symptoms in most others. Doses of 125 to 250 mg administered twice daily are recommended for prevention of AMS starting 24 to 48 hrs prior to ascent and continuing for 48 hrs after arrival. A 500-mg sustained-action capsule of acetazolamide is probably equally as effective but side effects may be more prominent with this dose. The U.S. Food and Drug Administration recommends 500 to 1,000 mg daily for prevention of AMS in a high-risk scenario (rapid ascent >3,000 m).

> **Acute Mountain Sickness**
> Key Points
> - Directly related to rate and magnitude of ascent.
> - *Everyone* is susceptible.
> - Predominant symptom is *headache*.
> - Prevent by staging, graded ascent, or acetazolamide.
> - Treat with descent, acetazolamide, dexamethasone, supplemental oxygen, hyperbaric bag, or combination therapy.
> - ***Do not ascend with AMS.***
> - Can evolve to HACE or HAPE.

Common side effects include taste alterations, numbness, tingling, or vibrating sensations in hands, feet, and lips, and ringing in the ears. Side effects subside after the medication is stopped. Acetazolamide is a sulfa drug and should not be used in sulfa-sensitive individuals.

(b) Dexamethasone (Decadron®), a corticosteroid, is also effective for prevention of AMS in sulfa-sensitive individuals or during short-duration military missions. Dexamethasone is given in 4 mg doses every 6 to 8 hrs starting 24 hrs prior to ascent and continuing for 48 hrs after arrival. Unlike acetazolamide, dexamethasone treats the symptoms of AMS caused by mild brain edema but does not aid acclimatization. Once dexamethasone is discontinued, rebound of AMS is likely. Soldiers taking dexamethasone should not ascend until they have demonstrated wellness off the steroid (for example, at least 12 hrs after the last dose). Potential side effects of dexamethasone include euphoria, trouble sleeping, and an increased blood sugar level in diabetics. The combination of acetazolamide and low-dose dexamethasone as a treatment for AMS may be superior to the use of acetazolamide alone. (Decadron® is a registered trademark of Merck and Company, Inc., Whitehouse Station, New Jersey.)

(c) There is no scientifically proven benefit to taking Ginkgo biloba or any other herbal supplement for the prevention of AMS or any other altitude illness.

(7) Treatment of AMS is based on the severity of symptoms (see table 6–4).

(a) The only sure treatment for AMS is descent to a lower elevation. A Soldier can descend by walking but should not be allowed to descend alone.

(b) Acute mountain sickness by itself does not mean that descent is absolutely necessary. Stopping the ascent to rest and acclimatize to the same altitude will resolve AMS in 3 days or less in most Soldiers. In cases of mild AMS, this is the best option.

(c) Medical therapy is crucial when descent is not possible. Acetazolamide in divided doses from 250 to 500 mg or one 500 mg extended-release capsule per day is the best choice for treating AMS. Dexamethasone in doses of 4 mg every 6 hrs will also treat AMS successfully. Symptoms of AMS often recur when dexamethasone is stopped. Soldiers who do not respond to medical therapy should descend to a lower altitude.

(d) Continuous moderate-flow supplemental oxygen (2 to 4 L/min by mask or nasal cannula) can be used to treat AMS. If pulse oximetry is available, oxygen can be titrated lower (1 to 2 L/min) to maintain $SaO_2 \geq 90$ percent. Oxygen is a precious commodity at high altitude and, as such, is usually reserved for more serious cases of HACE and HAPE.

(e) A portable hyperbaric chamber can be used to treat AMS (2 pounds per square inch (psi) for 2 to 4 hrs) (appendix G). Treatment with a hyperbaric chamber is essentially equivalent to descent (for example, 2,000 m lower elevation for every 2 psi of pressure) or treatment with oxygen. Supplemental oxygen can be provided by nasal cannual or mask to increase hyperbaric treatment efficacy.

(f) Specific symptoms of AMS can be treated with various palliative drugs. Care must be taken not to administer medications that could depress respiration or cognitive function. Analgesics for treating altitude headache include aspirin (325 to 1,000 mg every 4 to 6 hrs), acetaminophen (325 to 1,000 mg every 4 to 6 hrs, not to exceed 4,000 mg per day) and ibuprofen (200 to 800 mg every 4 to 6 hrs, not to exceed 3,200 mg per day) or other nonsteroidal anti-inflammatory drugs (NSAIDs) in the usual doses. The use of NSAIDs for AMS headache should be avoided or minimized during combat operations because of their detrimental effect on blood coagulation. Prochlorperazine (5 to 10 mg every 6 to 8 hrs) can be used to treat nausea and vomiting. Alcohol and sedative hypnotics should be avoided because of their depressive effect on respiration, especially during sleep. Zolpidem (10 mg) an hour before bedtime does not depress ventilation at altitude and may be used to treat insomnia in persons with AMS. Table 6–4 provides a complete listing of treatment and prevention options for AMS.

(8) The prognosis for AMS is good in that it normally resolves within 24 to 72 hrs without any adverse consequences. It resolves more rapidly with descent. Soldiers with AMS may have difficulty performing normal job duties and require duty limitations. Once symptoms resolve, Soldiers can return to full duty. Soldiers with persistent symptoms may require a temporary profile and should be considered for redeployment to lower altitude. Soldiers who, in spite of prophylactic measures, have recurrent or incapacitating episodes of AMS on repeat deployment to high altitude should be considered for a permanent physical profile to prevent their future deployment to mountain areas.

Table 6–4
Field treatment and prevention of acute mountain sickness

Severity	Treatment Options	Prevention
Mild	1. Descend 500 m or more. 2. Stop ascent, rest, and acclimatize at the same altitude. 3. Administer acetazolamide (125–250 mg twice daily, or 500 mg extended release) until symptoms improve. 4. Treat symptoms as necessary with analgesics and antiemetics. 5. Use a combination of therapies 1–4.	1. Staged and graded ascent. 2. Intermittent hypoxic exposure. 3. Avoid overexertion. 4. Take acetazolamide (125–250 mg twice daily or 500 mg extended release) 24 hrs before ascent and for 48 hrs after arrival. 5. Take dexamethasone (4 mg every 6 to 8 hrs) in short-duration military missions starting 24 hrs before ascent until mission cessation. 6. Consider a high carbohydrate diet.
Moderate	1. Descend 500 m or more. 2. Stop ascent, rest, and acclimatize at the same altitude. 3. Administer acetazolamide (125–250 mg twice daily or 500 mg extended release) until symptoms improve. 4. Administer dexamethasone (4 mg every 6 hrs). 5. Administer low-flow (1–2 L/min) or moderate-flow oxygen (2–4 L/min) to maintain oxygen saturation ≥90%. 6. Use a portable hyperbaric chamber at 2 psi for 2 to 4 hrs. 7. Use a combination of therapies 1–6.	1. Same as for *mild* AMS. 2. Treat *mild* AMS early to prevent progression to *moderate* AMS.

Severe	1. Immediately descend 500–1,000 m.
	2. If descent is not possible:
	  • Treat the same as *moderate* AMS.
	  • Monitor for progression to HACE or HAPE.
		1. Same as for *moderate* AMS.
		2. Treat *mild* or *moderate* AMS early to avoid progression to *severe* AMS.

b. *High altitude cerebral edema (HACE).*

(1) High altitude cerebral edema is a potentially fatal accumulation of fluid in brain tissue that occurs in Soldiers who rapidly ascend from low (<1,200 m) to high altitude (>2,500 m) or from high to higher altitude and stay there for a few days or more. The pathophysiology of HACE is thought to involve a hypoxia-induced vasogenic edema, in which protein-rich fluid spreads into the extracellular space through a compromised blood-brain barrier, or cytotoxic

edema, in which intracellular fluid accumulates in neurons and neuroglia, or a combination of both. High altitude cerebral edema is the more severe end of the spectrum of altitude-induced edema in the brain with subclinical cerebral edema manifested as AMS at the other end. High altitude cerebral edema can have a significant impact on military units operating at high altitude due to its serious prognosis and the need for rapid evacuation.

(2) The incidence of HACE is rare (usually less than 1 to 2 percent of persons going to high altitude). The magnitude of hypoxic stress is a major determinant of occurrence. While HACE can occur as low as 2,500 m, the vast majority of cases occur above 3,500 m, particularly with rapid ascent. Other contributory risk factors include the same risk factors as for AMS. Acute mountain sickness itself is considered a risk factor. Continued ascent by Soldiers with AMS carries a very high risk for development of HACE. A previous episode of HACE also confers a high risk for recurrence.

(3) Signs and symptoms of HACE are neurologic manifestations of progressive cerebral edema. A change in mental status (for example, confusion, disorientation, inability to talk coherently) and truncal ataxia (for example, swaying of the upper body, especially when walking) are hallmark characteristics of HACE. Early signs and symptoms resemble AMS and include severe headache, nausea, vomiting, and extreme lassitude. Headache, however, as well as other symptoms of AMS are not invariably present. Neurologically related changes such as visual abnormalities, numb or tingling parts of the body, bowel and bladder malfunction, hallucinations (visual and/or auditory) and seizures may occur. Soldiers may appear anxious, irritable, and withdrawn. Rapid pulse, cyanosis, and general pallor are commonly present. Those with HACE often have accompanying symptoms of HAPE (for example, dyspnea at rest, dry cough). The mean onset time of symptoms following ascent is 5 days with a range of 1 to 13 days. The later onset of HACE is thought to reflect the time for subclinical edema, initially manifested as AMS, to progress to clinically apparent HACE. Untreated, HACE can progress to coma in 12 hrs and death within 24 hrs, but the course can also be more fulminant with death occurring in less than 12 hrs.

(4) Diagnosis of HACE is based upon the presence of signs and symptoms of cerebral edema (text box) beginning within a few days to weeks in a setting of recent gain in altitude. Having the Soldier suspected of HACE perform a "tandem gait test" in which he or she is required to walk a straight line with one foot immediately in front of the other will aid diagnosis. Mental status can be assessed by questionnaire and observation. Because the early signs and symptoms are similar to AMS, medical personnel need to maintain a high index of suspicion for HACE in AMS victims.

> **Diagnosis of HACE**
> Key Points
> In the setting of a recent gain in altitude, either of the following signs/symptoms will be present:
> - The presence of a change in mental status and/or truncal ataxia in a person with AMS.
> - The presence of both mental status changes and truncal ataxia in a person without AMS.

Papilledema (that is, optic disc swelling) caused by increased intracranial pressure may be present in up to half of the Soldiers with HACE, but is not universal. If a lumbar puncture is performed, the cerebral spinal fluid pressure is elevated. Cerebral edema may be apparent on a computed tomography scan or magnetic resonance imaging of the brain.

(5) Differential diagnosis for HACE includes altitude-related stroke or transient ischemic attack (TIA), viral or bacterial infection, migraine cephalgia, trauma, hypothermia, hypohydration, hypoglycemia, substance abuse, psychosis and severe cerebral hypoxia resulting from HAPE. Symptoms suggestive of HACE in a setting of recent gain in altitude are probably due to HACE and should be treated as such until proven otherwise. All misdiagnoses must be eliminated by a physical exam, history, or treatment. Fever is usually absent in HACE, and alcohol, psychosis, or other drug use can be excluded by the history. Decreased body temperature may be indicative of hypothermia. Rest and rehydration can eliminate fatigue and hypohydration. Carbon monoxide poisoning can be excluded by history of recent exposure in a tent, cave or vehicle with a heater, stove or running motor. Check for signs of accompanying HAPE (for example, rales, dry cough, frothy pink or blood sputum) and, if present, treat for HAPE. Suspected HACE requires immediate therapeutic intervention requiring evacuation to a lower altitude.

(6) There is no definitive evidence for effective measures to prevent HACE because of its low incidence. Given the concept that AMS represents a mild form of HACE, the same prophylactic measures used to prevent AMS may also prevent HACE. Soldiers with AMS should not continue ascent.

(7) Treatment of HACE is immediate descent at the first sign of truncal ataxia or change in mental status. Do not delay descent while waiting for a helicopter. Delay may take a slightly confused, slightly ataxic Soldier to a condition of being comatose or unable to walk at all. The greater the descent, the better the outcome. Descent of 500 to 1,000 m may be required for clinical improvement, and descent to altitudes of less than 2,500 m is optimal. Affected Soldiers can descend by foot if they are ambulatory and are accompanied. In situations where descent is delayed by weather, tactical situation, or other contingency, onsite treatment can save a Soldier's life.

(a) Continuous supplemental oxygen at flow rates of 4 to 6 L/min by mask or nasal cannula for 4 to 6 hrs should be administered, but should not be used as a substitute for descent.

(b) Hyperbaric bag therapy (2 psi for 6 hrs) can save a Soldier's life but should not be used as a substitute for descent. Supplemental oxygen can be provided by nasal cannula or mask to increase treatment efficacy.

(c) Dexamethasone is the most widely accepted pharmacologic agent for treatment of HACE. It is administered in doses of 8 mg initially followed by 4 mg every 6 hrs. It should be continued until clinical signs of resolution are apparent.

(d) Furosemide, a loop diuretic, can be given in doses of 80 mg twice daily for a total of two doses. Careful attention must be paid to volume status when using potent diuretic agents.

High Altitude Cerebral Edema
Key Points
• Occurs most often at >3,500 m.
• Do not ascend with AMS present.
• Gait ataxia and mental confusion are the two hallmarks of HACE.
• **Immediate descent required for treatment.**
• If descent is not possible, supplemental oxygen or hyperbaric chamber can save a Soldier's life.
• Administer dexamethasone.
• Consider furosemide.

(e) Following descent, hospital management of HACE consists of supplemental oxygen (maintain arterial oxygen levels >90 percent), dexamethasone, supportive care, and possibly diuretic agents. Comatose Soldiers may require intubation and bladder catheterization. Consideration should be given to intubation with hyperventilation to reduce intracranial pressure in comatose Soldiers.

Table 6–5
Field treatment and prevention of high altitude cerebral edema

Symptoms	Treatment	Prevention
• Mental confusion • Ataxia • Severe lassitude	1. Descend **immediately** (500 to 1,000 m) until symptoms resolve. 2. If descent impossible— • Administer oxygen (4–6 L/min for 4–6 hrs). • Use a portable hyperbaric chamber at 2 psi for 6 hrs. • Administer dexamethasone, 8 mg intramuscularly initially, followed by 4 mg every 6 hrs. • Use a combination of therapies 1 and 2.	1. Staged and graded ascent. 2. Avoid direct ascent to >3,500 m. 3. Avoid overexertion. 4. Take acetazolamide (125 to 250 mg twice daily) 24 hrs before ascent and for 48 hrs after ascent. 5. Consider dexamethasone (4 mg every 6 to 8 hrs) in short-duration, high-risk missions 24 hrs before ascent until mission cessation. 6. **Do not ascend with symptoms of AMS.** 7. Treat AMS early.

(8) Prognosis for HACE is good if Soldiers are evacuated rapidly. If Soldiers are not evacuated rapidly, those who survive may have prolonged or permanent neurologic damage. Although mental status changes usually resolve fairly quickly, some ataxia may persist for days or weeks. Soldiers who survive should be evaluated for neurologic deficits that might affect their performance of military duties. Those with persistent neurologic deficits must be considered for an appropriate physical profile and possible Medical Evaluation Board (MEB). Soldiers who have had one episode of HACE are at increased risk of future episodes. Soldiers who have a repeat episode of HACE should be considered for a permanent physical profile to limit high altitude exposure.

c. High altitude pulmonary edema (HAPE).

(1) High altitude pulmonary edema is a noncardiogenic, potentially fatal accumulation of fluid in the lungs, which occurs in Soldiers that rapidly ascend from low (<1,200 m) to high altitude (>2,500 m) or from high to higher altitude and stay there for a few days or more. It also occurs in long-term high altitude residents who reascend rapidly to high altitude following a stay at low altitude lasting several weeks. The edema is caused by the combination of hypoxia-induced pulmonary vasoconstriction and increase in permeability of the pulmonary capillary

endothelium. The end result is overflow of fluid from the bloodstream into the lungs, hindering the normal exchange of gases between the lungs and circulating blood. Untreated, HAPE can be rapidly fatal (6 to 12 hrs) and is the most common cause of death among the altitude illness syndromes. It is often preceded by AMS and is frequently seen in individuals with HACE, but most cases of HAPE occur without concomitant HACE. Although the incidence of HAPE is relatively low, its impact on military units can be significant because of the serious prognosis and need for rapid evacuation.

(2) The incidence of HAPE depends on the altitude achieved, rate of ascent, and individual susceptibility (ranges from 2 to 15 percent of persons going to altitudes above 2,500 m). Other risk factors for HAPE include vigorous exercise, anxiety, young age, male gender, cold exposure, blunted ventilatory drive, recent upper respiratory tract infection, and preexisting medical conditions (that is, pulmonary hypertension). There is a high rate of recurrence (60 to 70 percent) in individuals who have had a prior episode of HAPE. The incidence of HAPE in long-term high altitude residents who return to altitude after a short stay (several weeks) at low altitude is as high as 20 percent. It is not uncommon for HAPE symptoms to start during the second night of sleep at altitude.

(3) Signs and symptoms of HAPE are related to the progressive pulmonary edema and resultant worsening hypoxemia. Early in the course, dyspnea at rest and a dry cough should raise suspicion of HAPE. Reduced exercise tolerance and chest tightness may also be present. Resting tachycardia and tachypnea greater than that induced by altitude alone may also be present. Soldier's nail beds and lips may be more cyanotic than other unit members at the same altitude. Crackles are evident on chest auscultation. Fever is common but rarely exceeds 38.3 °C. A mild increase in white blood cell count may be present with HAPE.

(a) As HAPE progresses, the cough may become productive with frothy and sometimes pink or blood-streaked sputum. Rales become more numerous and widespread, and wheezing may develop. Lung sounds may progress to an audible gurgling in the airway. Orthopnea may occur in some individuals (<20 percent). Progressive hypoxemia causes progressive dyspnea and cyanosis. Arterial blood gas measurements (if available) document significant hypoxemia, hypocapnia, and a slight increase in pH. Mental status deteriorates with progressive confusion and sometimes hallucinations. Ultimately, obtundation, coma and death will occur without treatment.

(b) When available, a chest x-ray will show multiple patchy interstitial or alveolar pulmonary infiltrates. The infiltrates may be predominant in the right middle lobe of the lung. The pulmonary vaculature may be widened, but the heart size is invariably normal. Electrocardiogram

> **Diagnosis of HAPE**
> Key Points
> In the setting of a recent gain in altitude, at least two of the following symptoms will be present:
> - Dyspnea at rest.
> - Cough.
> - Weakness or decreased exercise performance.
> - Chest tightness or congestion.
>
> At least two of the following signs will be present:
> - Crackles or wheezing in at least one lung.
> - Central cyanosis.
> - Tachpnea.
> - Tachycardia.

often shows a right strain pattern with rightward axis clockwise rotation, T-wave inversion in the precordial leads, an R-wave in leads V_{1-2}, and an S-wave in leads V_{5-6}.

(4) Diagnosis of HAPE is based upon the presence of signs and symptoms beginning within 24 to 72 hrs in a setting or recent gain in altitude. Treatment should be initiated immediately. Delay in treatment of progressive HAPE at high altitude usually results in death.

(5) Differential diagnosis of HAPE includes pneumonia, asthma, high altitude cough/bronchitis, congestive heart failure, myocardial infarction, mucus plugging, pulmonary embolus, and, in a military setting, possible exposure to chemical warfare agents. Until the 1960's, HAPE was often misdiagnosed as "pneumonia" due to the presence of fever and leukocytosis, and inappropriately treated with antibiotics. All misdiagnoses must be eliminated by a physical exam, history, or treatment. The diagnostic test to distinguish pneumonia from HAPE is descent; HAPE will improve rapidly but pneumonia will not. A history of symptoms prior to high altitude travel may indicate a preexisting medical condition such as asthma. Chronic, dry cough can occur at very high altitude (usually >4,500 m) due to irritation of the throat by breathing cold, dry air. High altitude cough is not associated with rales, sputum production, or desaturation with exercise. Pain with breathing may indicate a blood clot in the lungs while pain and swelling in the legs could indicate a blood clot in the legs. Soldiers with evolving HAPE may have normal oxygen saturations at rest. Always try to provoke desaturation in Soldiers suspected of having HAPE with a simple exercise test, which consists of walking 100 m on level ground at a reasonable pace to get out of breath. Soldiers with HAPE will desaturate more than Soldiers with simple fatigue or high altitude bronchitis.

(6) Prevention of HAPE includes staged and graded ascent, avoidance of risk factors, and pharmacologic prophylaxis. Adequate acclimatization can be achieved by limiting the ascent rate using the same graded ascent or staging schedules used for preventing AMS (figure 3–2, chapter 3). Because SaO_2 is lowest during sleep, unacclimatized Soldiers should sleep at as low an altitude as possible. "Climb high, sleep low" is a frequently repeated and useful adage that expresses this principle. Soldiers, especially those with a prior history of HAPE, should also avoid cold exposure and strenuous exertion until adequately acclimatized.

(a) Nifedipine may prevent HAPE from developing in Soldiers who have a history of prior episodes of HAPE. Nifedipine is administered in a 20 to 30 mg extended-release dose every 12 hrs beginning on the day of ascent and continuing for 3 days after ascent. Because hypotension is a possible side effect of this dose regimen, medical officers should consider administering a test dose or starting the regimen prior to ascent to avoid this effect during ascent. Nifedipine is not indicated for Soldiers without a history of HAPE or for those with no prior altitude experience. For those Soldiers, acetazolamide may help prevent AMS and provide some protection against HAPE.

(b) Recently, phosphodiesterase inhibitors, tadalafil (10 mg twice daily), and sildenafil (50 mg every 8 hrs) have been studied for the prevention of HAPE because of the pulmonary vasodilator effects associated with these medications. When started 24 hrs prior to ascent, these medications prevented HAPE in susceptible individuals. Prophylactic inhalation of a beta$_2$ (β_2)-adrenergic agonist, salmeterol (125 micrograms (μg) twice daily), also decreased the incidence of HAPE in susceptible persons. The use of phosphodiesterase inhibitors and inhaled ß$_2$-adrenergic agonists as prophylaxis against HAPE needs further study before definitive recommendations can be given.

(7) Treatment of HAPE depends to some degree on the severity of the illness. Immediate descent is the definitive treatment for HAPE. Supplemental oxygen should always be used, when available, during descent. Because physical exertion, cold, and anxiety can increase pulmonary artery pressure, descent should be passive and the Soldier should be kept warm. In the absence of a means of passive descent, Soldiers who are ambulatory may walk down slowly, but must be accompanied and their physical exertion kept to a minimum.

(a) Descending may not always be feasible owing to weather conditions, tactical situation, or other contingency. Mild cases of HAPE can often be successfully treated with bed rest and supplemental oxygen (2 to 4 L/min) for 48 to 72 hrs, but descent is still mandatory for all but mild cases. In the absence of supplemental oxygen, use of a hyperbaric chamber may be lifesaving but may require ≥4 hrs of treatment to be effective for HAPE. Use of positive end-expiration pressure delivered by means of a mask or pursed-lips breathing helps improve gas exchange and can be a temporary measure.

(b) Nifedipine, a calcium channel blocker, can reduce pulmonary pressure by as much as 30 percent in 30 min and is efficacious in treating Soldiers with HAPE. In established cases of HAPE, nifedipine therapy can be initiated by administering 10 mg initially, then 30 mg of extended-release formulation every 12 to 24 hrs until the pulmonary edema has resolved and SaO$_2$ has returned to normal. Nifedipine should not be used in lieu of descent, supplemental oxygen, or hyperbaric bag therapy, but is appropriately used in conjunction with each of these other therapies. Acetazolamide seems to be beneficial when given early in the course of HAPE because it prevents further impairment of pulmonary gas exchange.

High-Altitude Pulmonary Edema
Key Points

- Noncardiogenic pulmonary edema.
- Can progress rapidly (<12 hrs) to death.
- Usually begins 2 to 4 days after rapid ascent >2,500 m.
- Reduced exercise performance and dry cough are early hallmarks of HAPE.
- Young age, male sex, and strenuous exercise are high risk factors.
- Prevent by staging and graded ascent and nifedipine.
- Treat with descent, supplementary oxygen, hyperbaric chamber, nifedipine or combination.
- **Immediate descent is necessary in all but mild cases.**

Table 6–6
Field treatment and prevention of high altitude pulmonary edema

Severity of HAPE	Treatment	Prevention
Mild • Dyspnea on moderate exertion; may be able to perform light activity • Heartbeat per min: <110 • Breaths per min: <20	1. Descend 500–1,000 m by passive means. 2. Stop ascent, bed rest and acclimatize at the same altitude. 3. Administer moderate flow oxygen at 2–4 L/min for 4–6 hrs. Maintain oxygen saturation at >90%. 4. Use hyperbaric bag treatment (2 psi for 4 hrs). 5. Nifedipine (10 mg initially followed by 30 mg every 12 to 24 hrs). 6. Use a combination of therapies 1–5. 7. Consider acetazolamide (125–250 mg twice daily).	1. Staged and graded ascent. 2. Avoid overexertion. 3. Avoid cold exposure. 4. Avoid rapid ascent >2,500 m. 5. Administer nifedipine (30 mg every 24 hrs) 1 day prior to ascent and for 3 days after ascent. 6. Consider tadalafil (10 mg twice daily), sildenafil (50 mg every 8 hrs), and salmeterol (125 μg twice daily).
Moderate • Symptoms of dyspnea, weakness, fatigue with **mild** exertion; cannot perform light activity; headache with cough, dyspnea at rest • Heartbeats per min: 110–120 • Breaths per min: 20–30	1. Descend immediately (500–1,000 m) until symptoms resolve. 2. If descent is impossible, treat the same as mild HAPE except supplemental oxygen should be 4–6 L/min for 4–6 hrs.	1. Same as for **mild** HAPE. 2. Treat **mild** HAPE early to avoid progression to **moderate** HAPE.
Severe • Clouded consciousness, stupor or coma • Severe dyspnea, headache, weakness, nausea at rest • Loose, recurrent, productive cough • Wheezy, difficult respirations; obvious cyanosis • Heartbeats per min: >120 • Breaths per min: >30	1. Descend immediately (500–1,000 m) until symptoms resolve. 2. If descent impossible— • Treat the same as moderate HAPE. • Monitor for signs of HACE.	1. Same as for **moderate** HAPE. 2. Treat **mild & moderate** HAPE early to avoid progression to **severe** HAPE.

(8) The prognosis for HAPE is relatively good if recognized early and treated appropriately. It usually resolves rapidly and without permanent adverse consequences; however, Soldiers who have experienced a previous episode of HAPE have a high rate of recurrence. Soldiers who have had HAPE can return to duty when their pulmonary edema has resolved and their SaO_2 has increased appropriately. They should also be considered for prophylactic treatment with nifedipine on any subsequent high altitude deployments. Individuals who experience HAPE, with or without prophylactic treatment, should be evaluated for a permanent physical profile to limit high altitude exposure.

   d. *Altitude-induced peripheral edema (AIPE).*

   (1) Altitude-induced peripheral edema refers to edema of the face, extremities, or both during altitude exposure. Peripheral edema and facial edema are relatively common. If seen as an isolated finding without other symptoms of AMS, it is not considered AMS and is not a contraindication to ascent. The underlying cause of all of the altitude-related edemas, including AIPE, is hypoxia-induced leakage of small blood vessels due to activation of permeability mediators as well as increased blood flow and pressure in specific organs and tissues. Insufficient diuresis and natriuresis, changes in renal blood flow, and perturbations in the fluid-volume regulatory hormones due to hypoxia, exertion, or both also likely contribute. The condition is benign, but may cause Soldiers enough discomfort to degrade their performance to some degree.

   (2) The incidence of AIPE has not been well delineated, but it may be substantial even at lower altitudes. Reports of AIPE range from 16 percent in trekkers at 4,200 m to 70 percent in mountaineers at 4,559 m. Altitude-induced peripheral edema appears to be more common in women than men but is not thought to be related to menstrual cycle or oral contraceptives. It is also much more common in individuals with other altitude illnesses.

   (3) Signs and symptoms of AIPE include facial edema, prominent periorbital edema, and/or edema in the upper and lower extremities. It is associated with a weight gain of 4 to 6 kg, or as much as 6 percent of body weight. Facial edema may become apparent as creases left in the skin by sun goggles or headbands. Extremity edema may cause skin indentations left by rings, watch bands, gloves, or socks and boots.

   (4) Diagnosis of AIPE is based on the presence of signs and symptoms in the setting of a recent gain in altitude. The diagnosis can often be made by history alone because it tends to recur consistently with repeated ascents.

Altitude-Induced Peripheral Edema
Key Points

- Edema of face and hands with recent gain in altitude.
- Benign condition but incidence is substantial.
- Associated with weight gain.
- Tends to reoccur with repeated ascents.
- Presence should prompt evaluation for AMS, HACE, and HAPE.
- Prevent with acetazolamide.
- Treat with salt restriction and acetazolamide.
- Immediate descent is **NOT** necessary.

---

   (5) Differential diagnosis of AIPE includes causes of edema seen at sea level such as congestive heart failure or other cardiogenic edema, cirrhosis, renal failure, allergic reactions, and edema of the upper extremities caused by packstraps or binding by tight clothing. This latter

condition, often termed "packstrap edema," is common in both military operations and recreational hiking. Packstrap edema is identified by its resolution after the constriction is removed. Most of the conditions included in the differential diagnosis can be ruled out through clinical history and physical exam. Given that AIPE is associated with other forms of altitude illness, its presence should prompt an evaluation for AMS, HACE and HAPE.

(6) Prevention of AIPE involves salt restriction and the acetazolamide regimen used to prevent AMS. It can be treated successfully with mild diuretics (a 20 to 40 mg dose of furosemide or 250 mg of acetazolamide every 8 hrs for 3 doses) and salt restriction. As with most altitude illness syndromes, the definitive treatment is descent to a lower elevation.

(7) The prognosis for AIPE is relatively good if it is not associated with more menacing forms of altitude illness. Many untreated Soldiers remain edematous for the entire time they are above their "trigger" altitude but diurese rapidly when they return to lower elevations. Others may eventually diurese at high altitude as they acclimatize. Given the benign but predictably recurrent nature of this condition, Soldiers do not need to be medically restricted from high altitude.

e. High altitude retinal hemorrhage (HARH).

(1) High altitude retinal hemorrhage is patchy bleeding from the retinal blood vessels at high altitude. With increasing altitude, there is a precipitous drop in ocular oxygenation. As the level of oxygenation decreases, autoregulation causes observable dilation of retinal arteries and veins and an increase in retinal blood flow. At 5,300 m, retinal blood flow is more than double that at sea level. Increased blood flow causes retinal vessels to increase in diameter and appear engorged and tortuous. These changes progress with increasing altitude and may be prominent at extreme altitude. High altitude retinal hemorrhages are thought to result from blood pressure "surges" within the distended vessels that cause erratic patterns of bleeding. High altitude retinal hemorrhages occurring outside the macula are usually asymptomatic, self-limited, and resolve without sequelae; those occurring inside the macula, however, may cause a sudden loss of central vision.

(2) The incidence of HARHs varies directly with altitude. High altitude retinal hemorrhages are rare below 3,000 m. High altitude retinal hemorrhages occur in up to 30 percent of Soldiers at 4,267 m, in 50 to 60 percent at 5,486 m, and probably in 100 percent above 6,800 m. High altitude retinal hemorrhages may be more common in those with AMS. Strenuous exercise and blood pressure surges caused by forced Valsalva maneuvers during active climbing or defecating are also risk factors. Other possible predisposing factors include systemic hypertension, hemoconcentration, and blood hyperviscosity caused by fluid shifts and dehydration at altitude. These conditions may lead to increased coagulability and decreased

> **High Altitude Retinal Hemorrhage**
> Key Points
> - Patchy bleeding from retinal blood vessels.
> - Rare below 3,000 m but universal above 6,000 m.
> - Asymptomatic and self-limited when outside the macula.
> - Loss of central vision or dark spots when inside the macula.
> - Diagnosis by fundoscopic exam.
> - Immediate descent is **NOT** necessary when outside the macula.
> - Descent is necessary when hemorrhage is inside the macula.

oxygen transport, which could contribute to the pathogenesis of HARH. No association has been found with age and gender.

(3) Signs and symptoms of HARHs are usually unrecognized because they are asymptomatic. However, HARH into the macular area will cause blurred vision and a dark area or gap in the visual field.

(4) Diagnosis of HARH is by fundoscopic exam. Fundoscopic exam will show hyperemia and engorgement of the disc and increased tortuosity of retinal vessels. High altitude retinal hemorrhages appear as "splinter-type" and "flame-type" hemorrhages in the superficial layers of the retina, but hemorrhages in the deeper layers appear dark and rounded or as what are known as "dot-and-blot-type" hemorrhages. Multiple HARHs are common. The diagnosis can be made by observing the HARHs in conjunction with a recent gain in altitude.

(5) Differential diagnosis for HARH includes hemorrhage from vascular disease, diabetes mellitus, septic infarcts, or from hypoxia caused by cardiac or respiratory disease. Carbon monoxide poisoning has also been associated with HARH.

(6) Prevention and treatment of HARH involves descent. Because HARHs outside of the macula cause few symptoms and usually do not cause a significant permanent visual defect, descent is not necessary when HARHs outside of the macula are discovered. When a macular or vitreous HARH is diagnosed, descent is imperative to promote healing and prevent further hemorrhage. Hemodilution, which may decrease blood viscosity and coagulation in dehydrated Soldiers, has been reported as a treatment for HARH associated with visual decrement. Since HARH can be associated with AMS, it seems logical to follow the same guidelines that are used to prevent AMS.

(7) The prognosis for HARH occurring outside the macula is good. High altitude retinal hemorrhage usually resolves 2 to 8 weeks following descent to low altitude. It is advisable that Soldiers with previous *symptomatic* HARHs not return to high altitude because of the possibility that hemorrhage will recur to the same area. Physical profiling is not indicated for HARH outside the macular area.

  f. High altitude pharyngitis/bronchitis.

(1) High altitude pharyngitis/bronchitis (for example, Khumbu cough) is thought to be irritation of the mucosal lining of the respiratory passages due to an increased volume of cold, dry air moving across them from the hypoxia-induced increase in ventilation. Altitude-induced tachypnea aggravates the problem. Cold-induced vasomotor rhinitis, especially at night, stimulates mouth breathing and also aggravates the problem. Although desiccation of mucous membranes can lead to an increased number of upper respiratory infections, high altitude pharyngitis/bronchitis is seldom due to infection. The impact of high altitude pharyngitis/bronchitis on military operations is related primarily to the discomfort it causes to individual Soldiers.

> **High Altitude Pharyngitis/Bronchitis**
> Key Points
> - Chronic cough due to irritation of respiratory passages.
> - Common at altitudes above 5,500 m.
> - Wear a silk balaclava.
> - Treat with soothing lozenges and cough suppressant.
> - Descent is **NOT** necessary.

(2) The incidence of high altitude pharyngitis/bronchitis is frequent during prolonged stays (>2 weeks) at high altitude and is very common at altitudes over 5,500 m.

(3) Signs and symptoms of high altitude pharyngitis/bronchitis include sore throat, chronic cough and severe cough spasms provoked by exercise. Cough spasms can be severe enough to cause rib fractures.

(4) Diagnosis of high altitude pharyngitis/bronchitis in a high mountain environment relies solely on sign and symptoms.

(5) Differential diagnosis of high altitude pharyngitis/bronchitis includes HAPE. Desaturation with mild activity will occur with HAPE but not with high altitude pharyngitis/ bronchitis.

(6) There is no known prophylaxis for high altitude pharyngitis/bronchitis. Treatment of high altitude pharyngitis and bronchitis involves ample hydration, steam inhalation, hard candies or soothing lozenges and a mild cough suppressant. Soldiers can use a mask or a porous, breathable silk balaclava as a mouth covering to reduce respiratory heat and moisture loss. Decongestant nasal sprays may relieve cold-induced vasomotor rhinitis and lessen mouth breathing.

(7) The prognosis of high altitude pharyngitis/bronchitis is good. Although the symptoms of high altitude pharyngitis/bronchitis may be uncomfortable and irritating, Soldiers seldom require duty limitations. Uncontrollable high altitude cough may present a security risk during covert operations.

g. Sleep disturbances.

(1) Periodic or Cheyne-Stokes breathing (alternating cycle of hyperpnea and apnea) during sleep is common at high altitude. The phenomenon is thought to be caused by a sleep-induced decrease in cortical influence on respiration combined with changes in the gain and sensitivity of the peripheral chemoreceptors, so that there is overcompensation for the altitude-induced hypoxemia. Increased ventilation lowers CO_2 enough to cause a hypocapnic apnea. The prolonged period of apnea (10 to 20 seconds without a breath are not unusual) can be particularly disturbing to Soldiers who observe them in their companions. The periods of apnea can cause profound reductions in oxygen saturation. At an altitude of 5,500 m, the average reduction can amount to 10 percent. This additional reduction in SaO_2 is associated with large performance decrements while awake and may exacerbate altitude illness symptoms upon awakening. Sleep architecture is also fragmented at high altitude with frequent short arousals and less time spent in "deep" or "slow-wave" sleep (stages 3 and 4) and rapid eye movement (REM) sleep. Although the arousals are short enough that they may not be noticed by a nonsleeping observer, they are very apparent to the Soldier attempting to sleep. Reports of "not being able to sleep" and "awake half the night" are common. Frequent arousals may contribute to mood changes and daytime symptoms of somnolence.

> **Sleep Disturbances**
> Key Points
> - Alternating periods of fast breathing and breath holding.
> - Occurs in nearly everyone above 3,000 m.
> - Vivid dreams, mood changes, and daytime fatigue are common.
> - Treat with supplemental oxygen and acetazolamide.
> - Descent is **NOT** necessary.

(2) The incidence of periodic breathing during sleep at altitude is high. Periodic breathing during sleep occurs in nearly everyone above 3,000 m and is universal above 6,000 m. However, sleep disturbances have been reported as low as 1,500 m.

(3) The signs and symptoms caused by periodic breathing at altitude are vivid dreams or nightmares, a feeling of poor or unrefreshing sleep, mood changes, a sensation of suffocation, or a feeling of not having slept much at all. Daytime fatigue is common.

(4) The diagnosis of periodic breathing at altitude is made by noting the signs and symptoms of disordered sleep in a Soldier who has recently ascended to moderate or high altitude or at any time at very high and extreme altitudes.

(5) The differential diagnosis of periodic breathing at altitude include other possible causes of poor sleep in Soldiers deployed to high altitude (for example, cold, unfamiliar bedding or sleeping surface, crowded sleeping quarters, jet lag). Preexisting pathological sleep disorders, such as Cheyne-Stokes respiration in chronic heart failure and obstructive sleep apnea syndrome, can be identified by a complete clinical history.

(6) The most reliable method to treat disordered sleep at altitude is to raise inspired oxygen by descending in elevation. Descent below 2,500 m will reduce altitude-induced sleep problems for the vast majority of Soldiers. When descent is not possible, inspired oxygen levels can be raised using low-flow (1 to 2 L/min) supplemental oxygen during sleep. However, the logistics of supplying even low-flow oxygen to Soldiers in an operational setting will often be prohibitive. Acetazolamide is the treatment of choice for sleep disturbances at high altitude if descent is not possible and has the added advantage of being an effective prophylactic against AMS. Individuals using acetazolamide for AMS prophylaxis require no additional dosage for improving sleep, while those not on the medication can use 125 or 250 mg once nightly prior to sleep. The combination of 10 mg temazepam and 500 mg acetazolamide 1 hr before bedtime is also effective in improving sleep and maintaining oxygen saturation. Inappropriate treatment of altitude-induced sleep problems solely with hypnotic drugs (that is, sleeping pills) can exacerbate hypoxemia due to depression of ventilation.

(7) Altitude-induced sleep problems resolve on their own upon return to sea level, and there appear to be no long-lasting sequale. Strong consideration should be given to treating all military personnel deployed to mountain environments above 3,000 m in order to prevent altitude-induced sleep problems during the initial ascent. At altitudes under 5,000 m, treatment can be discontinued for most individuals as they successfully acclimatize. There is no need for Soldiers to be put on physical profile for altitude-related sleep problems unless their job duties require sustained vigilance.

h. Blood-clotting disorders.

(1) Intravascular blood-clotting (thromboembolic) disorders and minor bleeding phenomena occur frequently at high altitude which suggests a possible altitude-induced disruption of normal hemostatis mechanisms. Thromboembolic events include thrombophlebitis, deep venous thrombosis (DVT), pulmonary embolism, TIAs, and stroke in healthy, young Soldiers who do not ordinarily develop such catastrophic problems. With the exception of thrombophlebitis, these events are relatively rare, but can have a significant impact on military operations due to the requirement to evacuate the affected Soldier. Possible causes for these phenomena include hypoxia-induced polycythemia and clotting abnormalities, but also include environmental and

mission-related factors such as dehydration and cold and venous stasis caused by prolonged periods of inactivity and/or by constriction from tight-fitting clothing or equipment.

(2) The incidence of altitude-related thromboembolic events is rare below 4,300 m. At altitudes >4,300 m, these events are not uncommon, and thrombophlebitis appears to be relatively common.

(3) The signs and symptoms of altitude-related thromboembolic events are the same as those that occur at low altitude and include—

(a) Pain, swelling and warmth in the affected limb from a peripheral venous thrombi.

(b) Chest pain, dyspnea, hypoxemia, cough and hemoptysis from a pulmonary emboli.

(c) Transient or permanent, focal or global neurological abnormalities, coma or death in the case of a cerebral thrombi.

(4) Diagnosis of thromboembolic disease in a high mountain environment relies solely on sign and symptoms. If the Soldier can be evacuated to appropriate facilities, standard methods (for example, Doppler ultrasound, roentgenography, angiography) can be used to confirm the diagnosis.

(5) Differential diagnosis for thromboembolic events must include other altitude-related conditions that can have similar manifestations. Cellulitis, HACE, and HAPE can cause signs and symptoms similar to those of thromboembolism.

(6) Prevention of altitude-related thromboembolic events relies on reducing the risk factors by maintaining adequate hydration and warmth and by avoiding conditions that might cause venous stasis. Although aspirin has been suggested as a preventative treatment for altitude-related thromboembolic events, it has not been studied. The risk of side effects, including an increase in retinal hemorrhages or other altitude-related bleeding, may make aspirin unsuitable for prophylaxis at altitude. With the possible exception of mild, superficial thrombophlebitis, the occurrence of an altitude-related thromboembolic event mandates a rapid evacuation to medical facilities at a lower altitude. Treatment at medical facilities follows standard clinical guidelines, including appropriate anticoagulation. In a field setting, low-dose subcutaneous heparin (5,000 units every 8 to 12 hrs) can be used for anticoagulation.

(7) The prognosis for thromboembolic events occurring at high altitude is the same as at sea level, assuming that the Soldier can be evacuated for treatment in a timely fashion. Mortality and morbidity are very high if the Soldier remains at high altitude without treatment. The limitations on return to duty include the necessity for prolonged anticoagulant therapy, neurological deficits from stroke, and decreased lung function from pulmonary emboli. The incidence of recurrent thromboembolic events during subsequent altitude exposure in Soldiers who have had a previous event in the mountains is not known. Presumably, Soldiers with a preexisting coagulopathy would be at increased risk. Therefore,

| **Blood-clotting Disorders** |
| Key Points |
| • Disruption of normal hemostatis at altitude which causes blood clots. |
| • Swelling of a vein due to blood clots is common. |
| • Pain, swelling, and warmth in the affected limb. |
| • Maintain adequate hydration and warmth. |
| • **Immediate evacuation** is required except for mild, superficial vein swelling. |

military members with a previous history of thromboembolic phenomenon at high altitude should probably be restricted from deployment to the mountains to limit potential impact of a recurrent event.

i. Subacute mountain sickness. Subacute mountain sickness is a syndrome of persistent symptoms which may occur in some Soldiers during prolonged deployment (weeks to months) to elevations about 3,500 m. Common manifestations include sleep disturbances, anorexia, weight loss, daytime somnolence and subnormal mentation. The condition reflects a failure to acclimatize adequately. Some relief from symptoms can be obtained with low-flow oxygen and acetazolamide, but there are no other means to accelerate or insure acclimatization in these Soldiers. They should be returned to low altitude as soon as practical. Soldiers who experience subacute mountain sickness may have subtle physiologic abnormalities that will consistently limit their ability to adequately acclimatize. A permanent physical profile should be considered to limit their altitude exposure.

j. Immune system suppression. High altitude has been shown to degrade immune function in experimental conditions due to altitude-induced increases in adrenal corticosteroid hormone levels. Exposure to high altitude for prolonged periods can depress cell-mediated immunity but seems to have little effect on humoral immune function. Effects on cell-mediated immunity include—

(1) A decreased ability for in vitro monocyte activation despite an increase in monocyte numbers.

(2) A decrease in measures of natural cell cytotoxicity. Measures of humoral immune function, including serum immunoglobulin levels and B cell response to vaccination with T-cell independent antigen, are not affected by high altitude.

k. Poor wound healing. Superficial wounds heal slowly at altitudes greater than 5,000 m. The combination of low tissue SaO_2 and cold temperatures might decrease the circulation in the extremities enough to slow healing of wounds. The incidence of immune system suppression at high altitude is unknown. Clinical importance of altitude-induced immune suppression appears limited to an increase in skin infections and cellulitis that may not respond well to treatment while the patient remains at high altitude. Diagnosis of poor wound healing in a high mountain environment relies solely on signs and symptoms. The prudent course is to evacuate wounded Soldiers to low altitude or provide them with supplemental oxygen therapy. Soldiers seldom require duty limitations once the infection or wound is healed.

6–3. Environmental/mission factor threats

a. Introduction. In high mountain areas, environmental and mission factors other than hypobaric hypoxia can cause medical problems in military personnel. These factors include trauma, climatic conditions, solar radiation, lightning strikes, CO poisoning, dehydration, negative energy balance, poor sanitation, and hemorrhoids. In many instances, these problems may be far more clinically significant than those caused by hypoxia itself (for example, lightning strike will cause more disability than HARH). Often these problems will be more frequent than hypoxia-related problems (for example, cold injuries outnumber cases of HACE). Many of these problems, however, can be minimized or even eliminated by detailed planning and training prior to deployment as outlined in appendices H and I. Unlike hypobaric hypoxia, these factors are not unique to the high mountain environment and cause medical problems in other environments as well. Military medical personnel are often familiar with these medical problems because they have encountered them frequently. Therefore, these medical problems are not presented here in the same detail as the previous discussion of hypobaric-hypoxia-related problems. See appendix A for publications (for example, technical bulletins and field manuals) containing more detailed information about medical problems related to environmental and mission factors at high altitude.

  b. *Trauma.*

  (1) Trauma is common in the mountainous environment. The combination of rugged topography with hypoxia-impaired judgment and reasoning abilities is a major contributing factor to traumatic injury. The two most common injuries that affected infantry troops operating in Afghanistan were orthopedic injuries and low back injuries. Increased frequency of overuse injuries will often occur at the beginning of mountain operations due to changes in the biomechanics of marching and other activities caused by rugged, sloped terrain. If there is a significant component of technical climbing involved in the mission, upper extremity and especially finger injuries may be prominent. Current equipment and operating procedures for the U.S. Army dictate that Soldiers must wear full body armor even when conducting foot patrols over arduous terrain. This extra weight, situated on the torso, is cumbersome when navigating more difficult terrain where both hands and feet are required for movement. Snow, rain, and ice make footing and handholds more tenuous than when the weather is dry. Owing to steep terrain, falls are a major contributor to the tally of traumatic injuries. Mountaineering equipment with sharp points and surfaces, as well as military weapons, can cause lacerations and penetrating injuries during a long fall. Mountains can inflict trauma directly through rockslides and avalanches. Avalanches and rockslides often bury individuals, causing crush injury and asphyxiation.

  (2) Diagnosis, prevention, treatment and prognosis of trauma in mountain terrain follows standard clinical guidelines. Prevention of trauma in mountain terrain requires appropriate training and equipment. Training should include proper use of equipment such as crampons, ice axes, and climbing harnesses. Use of hiking sticks seems to prevent falls during recreational hiking. Soldiers should be familiarized with relevant environmental hazards such as avalanches and rockslides and know how to avoid being caught in them. Good physical conditioning helps to prevent accidents in the mountains by lessening the fatigue and lack of strength that contribute to accidents. Treatment options for trauma at high altitude may be limited by lack of specialized medical equipment in the field. Injured Soldiers may require evacuation to higher echelons for definitive medical care. Rest of the affected extremity is a prominent element of treatment. Most overuse injuries recover with time, but affected Soldiers may require a temporary physical profile consisting of minor duty limitations. Medical personnel must be mindful that the victim of trauma at altitude already has compromised oxygen delivery and likely decreased blood volume. These factors may precipitate development of shock.

  c. *Cold injury.*

  (1) Cold injuries are very common at high altitude. Once a Soldier has acclimatized to altitude, the incidence of hypoxia-related illness declines, and cold injuries are often the most common environmental injury. The full spectrum of cold injuries from hypothermia to freezing

and nonfreezing tissue injury can occur. At high altitude, mean ambient temperature drops approximately 2 to 6 °C for each 1,000-m increase in elevation. Progressively lower temperatures combined with high winds and precipitation, frequent components of mountain weather, can quickly lead to hypothermia. At the same time, the effects of hypobaric hypoxia on the body and on psychological function increase vulnerability in the cold. Altitude-induced increases in RBC mass and peripheral vasoconstriction from decreased plasma volume and dehydration significantly increase the risk of frostbite or freezing injury. Hypoxia-related errors in judgment and blunted reasoning ability hinder the normal behaviors that protect against cold stress. One of the most common scenarios in the mountains is that of climbers taking off their gloves and, owing to hypoxia, forgetting to put them back on thereby causing severe freezing injuries to their hands.

(2) Diagnosis, prevention, treatment, and prognosis of cold injuries in the mountains is the same as at low altitude and is described in TB MED 508 (see appendix A). Prevention of cold injury is the responsibility of the unit commander and the individual Soldier. It is based on planning, training, adequate hydration and nourishment, and protection afforded by protective clothing and shelter. Medical officers supporting units deployed to high altitude areas must be prepared to advise the commander on cold injuries and participate in appropriate planning and training of unit Soldiers.

d. Heat injury.

(1) Heat injury is much less common than cold injury in the mountains, but it does occur in certain situations. In fact, heat exhaustion was the fourth most common illness among Soldiers deployed to Afghanistan. Heat injury is usually due to a combination of factors that increase an individual's heat load. In high mountain environments, the most common factors are increased solar load due to lack of shade above timberline; increased light reflection off of rock, snow, and ice surfaces; dehydration, and increased metabolic heat production due to the increased physical effort needed to accomplish work while hypoxic. Heat exhaustion due to these conditions is often referred to as "glacier lassiture" and has been chronicled during climbing expeditions for many years.

(2) Diagnosis, prevention, treatment, and prognosis of heat injuries in the mountains is the same as at low altitude and is described in TB MED 507/AFPAM 48–152(I) (see appendix A). Because hypoxia does not appear to make a significant contribution to the pathophysiology of heat injury, there is no reason to believe that descent or the provision of supplemental oxygen would be of any significant benefit in treating heat injury itself. Medical officers supporting units deployed to high altitude areas must be prepared to advise the commander on heat injuries and participate in appropriate planning and training of unit Soldiers.

e. Solar radiation injury.

(1) Introduction. Excessive ultraviolet (UV) radiation from sunlight is a serious threat to military personnel operating in high mountain regions during daylight hours because several factors increase its damaging potential. The decreased UV filtering by the thinner atmosphere at high altitude causes an increased intensity of exposure (~ 4 percent for every 300 m) and a shift of the UV spectrum to more harmful shortwave lengths. Reflection from snow and ice increase the intensity of exposure (~75 percent of the incident radiation is reflected). Ultraviolet exposure can cause significant short-term disability to military personnel through severe sunburn and snow

blindness (solar keratitis). Ultraviolet exposure can also cause discomfort through mild sunburn and reactivation of cold sores on the lips. Diagnosis, prevention, treatment, and prognosis of solar radiation injuries is the same as at low altitude and is covered in Textbooks of Military Medicine: Medical Aspects of Harsh Environments, Volume 2, pages 815–853 (Rock and Mader 2002).

(2) Sunburn. Sunburn can occur with a much shorter exposure at high altitude and can be severe. Because people at high altitude are usually well-clothed for protection from the cold temperatures, the sunburn is often confined to the exposed skin of the face, especially the nose and lips. In areas of the mountains where the ambient temperatures are warmer, hiking or working in short pants can cause burns to the extremities and torso. Sunburn may be more likely to occur on partly cloudy or overcast days because Soldiers may not be aware of the threat and may not take appropriate precautions.

(a) Soldiers vary greatly in their risk for sunburn based on their skin type and pigment. Limiting skin exposure with clothes and sunscreen (sun protection factor (SPF) 15 and above) will prevent most sunburns. Application to skin areas that are normally shaded, such as the eyelids and under the chin, is necessary to reduce the likelihood of sunburn from light reflected off snow and rocks. Opaque agents, such as zinc oxide, red veterinary petrolatum or titanium dioxide, can be used for high-risk body areas such as the nose, lips, and tops of the ears. The agents should be used carefully in a tactical situation where they could make a Soldier more visible to opposing forces.

(b) Treatment for sunburn includes symptomatic relief with cold compresses. Topical anesthetics may cause sensitization and should be avoided. Ointments and creams containing antihistamines, steroids, and NSAIDs may be helpful, but have not been adequately studied. Aggressive treatment with systemic corticosteroids may be considered for severe sunburn over large areas of the body. Time for convalescence and any necessary duty restriction for sunburn depends upon the severity and extent of skin involved.

(3) Snow blindness. Snow blindness results when solar radiation "sunburns" the eyes. Eyes may feel painful and gritty, and there may be tearing, blurred vision, severe light sensitivity, and headache. Snow blindness can occur in a few hours of exposure, and there is no sensation of abnormality other than brightness as a warning that eye damage is occurring.

(a) Symptoms are maximal 6 to 8 hrs after exposure and resolve in 48 to 72 hrs. The use of eyewear or goggles that block more than 90 percent of UV radiation will help prevent snow blindness. To prevent injury from reflected light, protective eyewear should have side shields. Additionally, the eyewear should have a safety cord or strap to prevent its being lost accidentally. If sunglasses are not available, opaque eye covering (for example, tape-covered eyeglasses) with narrow horizontal slits provide adequate field-expedient eye protection.

(b) Treating snowblindness involves patching the eye and controlling the pain. Dilating the pupil and using ocular antibiotics are helpful. Pain control may require oral analgesics, sedatives, or both. The prognosis is generally good, although snow blindness may take several days to resolve, and the pain and visual decrements will require temporary, but significant, duty limitations. In severe cases, permanent damage can occur.

(4) Cold sores. Cold sores on the lips due to reactivation of latent herpes simplex virus infection by UV light is a common and well-known phenomenon at high altitude. Lesions can be treated with local application of an antiviral ointment such as acyclovir. There is probably

little utility in treating with an oral antiviral medication. Prevention of UV exposure using lip balms containing sunscreen protection (*para*-aminobenzoic acid (PABA)) and zinc oxide is generally effective in preventing cold sores at altitude. Prophylactic use of this treatment should be encouraged since these problems are preventable.

f. Lightning strikes.

(1) Lightning strikes are a significant seasonal hazard in the mountains, especially in exposed areas above timberline. The thunderstorms that generate lightning are more frequent over high mountains, and many people are killed or injured by lightning in mountain regions.

(a) Lightning can strike a person in several ways. It can strike a person directly or strike an object that the person is touching or holding. Direct strikes tend to cause the most severe injuries. Lightning can also jump from a nearby object that has been struck (that is, splash) or travel through the ground or water (that is, step voltage). These indirect strikes are less severe than the direct ones.

(b) Lightning injuries differ from electrical injuries caused by high voltage wires because the duration of exposure with lightning is so short that the current tends to "flashover" the body causing superficial burns rather than internal injury. "Fern-like" burns on the skin are characteristic of lightning strikes, but other types of burns often occur. Fatal injuries occur in only about one-third of personnel directly struck by lightning and usually result from prolonged respiratory, cardiac or combined cardiopulmonary arrest. All strikes can cause blunt trauma if the person struck is thrown by violent muscle contraction or falls while unconscious. Confusion and various neurologic abnormalities are universal sequelae of lightning strikes. Tympanic membrane rupture is so common as to be pathognomonic. Ocular injuries are also common, and many individuals develop cataracts within a few days of being struck.

(2) Prevention of lightning strikes depends upon avoiding areas where the risk is increased and taking appropriate protective action when those areas cannot be avoided. If caught in a lightning storm, seek a location with nearby projections or masses that are significantly higher than your head. In a forest, the best place is among shorter trees. Along a ridge, the preferable location is in the middle as the ends are more exposed and susceptible to strikes.

(a) Protective measures include taking shelter in solid-roofed structures or vehicles (tents and canvas-topped vehicles are not safe) because the strike will flow over the outer surface of the structure or vehicle. The recommended protective position in open terrain is crouching in a low spot with feet and legs pressed together to occupy as small an area as possible. If possible, sit on insulated objects such as a coiled rope, sleeping bag, or ensolite sleeping pad.

(b) Personal protection includes staying at least 5 m away from tall and large metal objects and from electrical and communication equipment. Portable radio-communications equipment with aerials are especially dangerous and should not be operated or carried during storms. Command posts and other areas where several Soldiers stand close together are also at high risk for step voltage, and Soldiers in these areas should spread out and crouch low to the ground.

(3) Treatment of lightning strikes involves immediate cardiopulmonary resuscitation if Soldiers are in arrest. Because most lightning victims who are not in immediate cardiopulmonary arrest do not progress to arrest, and many who are in arrest will recover spontaneously if supported, the normal triage should be reversed so that immediate care goes to the apparently "dead" victim. Cardiac activity tends to recover much more quickly than

respiratory function, so care should be taken to insure adequate ventilation. Trauma and burns caused by lightning can be treated using standard clinical guidelines. The prognosis for victims of lightning strikes who survive is good, initially, but after they recover from their acute injuries, victims may experience long-term effects, including posttraumatic stress disorder and other neuropsychological symptoms such as sleep and memory difficulties. Victims with permanent neurologic damage should be referred to an MEB.

g. Carbon monoxide poisoning.

(1) Carbon monoxide is a poisonous gas that cannot be seen or smelled. Carbon monoxide binds to red cells more readily than oxygen, so less oxygen is available to vital organs and tissues. Carbon monoxide is contained in the exhaust from stoves and vehicles. Carbon monoxide poisoning is a frequent environmental hazard during military operations at high altitude for at least two reasons—

(a) Inefficient fuel combustion caused by the low oxygen content of the air produces more CO than is produced by combustion at low altitude.

(b) Soldiers often run stoves, combustion heaters, and engines in enclosed, poorly ventilated spaces (for example, tents, caves, and vehicles) to avoid cold conditions outside. At high altitude, where the amount of oxygen in the blood is already limited, it takes less CO to cause more significant tissue hypoxia than at lower altitude. Early signs of CO poisoning include headache, nausea, malaise, and shortness of breath, which can progress to coma. High altitude retinal hemorrhages are also seen in CO poisoning. CO poisoning can cause a non-cardiogenic pulmonary edema similar to HAPE. Persons found unconscious in a closed tent or vehicle may be victims of CO poisoning, especially if the lips and skin are bright cherry red.

(2) Carbon monoxide poisoning can be prevented by maintaining adequate ventilation. Tents must not be airtight. Soldiers must not remain in stationary idling vehicles for long periods. Under no circumstances should a Soldier sleep in an idling vehicle. Occupants of idling vehicles should ensure that exhaust pipes are not blocked by snowbanks and that the windows of the vehicle are slightly opened. Work heaters in tents should be closely monitored to ensure that equipment is operating at maximum efficiency. Only U.S. Army-approved heaters (space heater Arctic, National Stock Number (NSN) 4520-01-444-2375; space heater small NSN 4520-01-478-9207; space heater medium, NSN 4520-01-329-3451; space heater convective, NSN 4520-01-431-8927) will be used. Only properly trained Soldiers will be permitted to set up, light, refuel, and maintain stoves. Stovepipes must be kept clean and must be tall enough to draft properly. A fire guard must be posted at all times. The tent doorway must be kept clear to allow easy escape in case of fire.

(3) The initial treatment for CO poisoning is to prevent further exposure by removing the source of CO or removing the patient from the source. Treatment then is similar to that at low altitude and consists of 100 percent oxygen and providing supportive care. Forced hyperventilation, especially with supplemental oxygen administered by a tight-fitting mask, will accelerate elimination of CO from the body. Since descent in elevation increases oxygen pressure, it is helpful to evacuate the patient to a lower altitude. Use of the hyperbaric chamber with supplemental oxygen is helpful when evacuation is prevented by weather or tactical situation. Soldiers who recover without neurological damage can return to high altitude duty without limitation. Those with significant sequelae will require physical profile or referral to an MEB based upon their condition.

h. Infectious diseases.

(1) Although there is some decrease in T-cell function at high elevations (see paragraph 6–2*j*), the patterns of infectious disease seen in high mountain areas primarily reflect patterns of exposure rather than any degree of immunodeficiency. In general, there are progressively fewer bacteria in the environment and fewer insect vectors at higher altitudes. This results in a more narrow spectrum of infectious disease at very high and extreme altitudes. The types of infections found there tend to be from endogenous bacterial flora and agents that are easily transmitted directly from person to person. Person-to-person transmission is enhanced by the tendency for Soldiers to crowd together in relatively small confined spaces (tents, vehicles, etc.) for relief from the cold. Sleeping toe to head limits exposure. Poor field sanitary conditions also increase exposure to infectious diseases at high altitude. Soldiers may not practice proper field sanitation or personal hygiene at very high altitudes due to the cold conditions, water shortage and hypoxia-induced decrements in energy and motivation. Commanders and medical personnel should insist that good personal hygiene and proper sanitation are accomplished.

(2) The spectrum of infectious diseases seen at moderate altitude is generally wider than at higher elevations. Insect-borne disease is more common with ticks and flies being significant vectors. In a few specific areas, malaria-bearing mosquitoes range as high as 1,829 m. Indigenous populations in mountain regions are another source of infectious disease because they tend to have generally poor economic status with limited or nonexistent public health systems. The problem is even more pronounced with refugees. High exposure rates to tuberculosis, hepatitis and diarrheal disease should be expected when Soldiers contact either refugees or indigenous populations.

(3) Travelers' diarrhea is strikingly common. Diarrhea was the third most common complaint among infantry deployed to the high mountains of Afghanistan. Travelers' diarrhea is defined as the occurrence of three or more unformed stools within a 24-hr period or any number of such unformed stools when accompanied by nausea, vomiting, abdominal cramps, or fever. The primary cause of travelers' diarrhea is infectious agents. Ingestion of contaminated food and water is thought to be the most common means of transmission of travelers' diarrhea. Soldiers should wash their hands before eating and avoid consuming untreated water, rice beer, raw vegetables, uncooked fish or meat, unpeeled fruit, cheese, ice cream or any kind of street vendor food. Filter, treat with chlorine or iodine, or boil all surface water.

(4) Travelers' diarrhea is a self-limited illness that will usually resolve on its own. Travelers' diarrhea falls into two main groups: presumed bacterial and presumed protozoal.

(a) The preferred treatment for bacterial diarrhea is one of the fluoroquinolone antibiotics such as norfloxacin, 400 mg twice daily for 3 days, or ciprofloxacin, 500 mg twice daily for 3 days. Giardia lamblis is a one-celled parasite that causes protozoal diarrhea and gastrointestinal upset. Protozoal diarrhea has a much longer incubation time than bacterial diarrhea, with onset of symptoms 10 to 14 days after ingestion.

(b) The preferred treatment for Giardia is tinidazole (2 g at bedtime for 2 nights) or metronidazole (500 mg 3 times a day for 7 days). A definitive diagnosis is made by identifying cysts in the stool or upper intestinal tract secretions. These regimens provide approximately an

80-percent cure rate and can be repeated, or a combination of these drugs can be used when the condition persists. While taking metronidazole, alcohol should be avoided until 24 hrs after last dose.

(c) There are several anti-motility medications that many trekkers carry and use against diarrhea, often with the mistaken impression that they are antibiotics. These medications slow transit time through the stomach (thus slowing diarrhea) but do not treat the infection. Medications such as diphenoxylate and loperamide are useful to treat cramping but should not be used without antibiotics to treat diarrhea. Diagnosis and treatment of infectious diseases at high altitude are the same as at low altitude and rely on antibiotics, supportive care, or both.

i. Negative fluid balance (dehydration).

(1) Negative fluid balance at high altitude is the result of fluid intake inadequate to compensate for the high rate of fluid loss. At high altitude, hypohydration is almost universal, and it degrades performance and contributes to various environmental injuries. Several factors increase fluid loss at high altitudes. The increased breathing at high altitudes causes increased water loss in the exhaled air, and the low ambient humidity, common to high altitude environments, causes greater water loss through evaporation of sweat from the skin. Additional sources of fluid loss include hypoxia-induced diuresis and vomiting associated with AMS. In addition to higher rates of fluid loss, fluid intake is also decreased at high altitude. Soldiers with AMS may voluntarily restrict fluids to minimize the severity of gastrointestinal distress. Decreased fluid intake due to hypoxia-induced blunting of thirst sensation and the difficulty of obtaining and transporting potable water may also contribute to dehydration. Hypoxia-induced malaise effect on judgment and reasoning can further limit intake. Additionally, a conscious decision may be made to limit water intake to avoid having to remove clothing to urinate in cold weather and dangerously rugged terrain.

(2) Diagnosis, prevention, treatment and prognosis of hypohydration is covered in TB MED 507/AFPAM 48–152(I). Diagnosis of hypohydration in a high altitude setting is somewhat complicated, because many of the common signs and symptoms of hypohydration (for example, malaise, dizziness, tachycardia, headache) could be due to hypobaric hypoxia or AMS. Facilities for laboratory evaluation to support a diagnosis are seldom available. The best advice for diagnosing hypohydration is monitoring urine color. If the urine color is turning deep yellow, orange or brown, suspect hypohydration. The best prevention for hypohydration is having water easily accessible. Supplementing the water with sports drinks (that is, Gatorade®) or similar electrolyte drinks will make the drinks more palatable, and the Soldiers will be more likely to consume those drinks. Soups with breakfast and dinner will also aid with water and mineral repletion. (Gatorade® is a registered trademark of Stokely-Van Camp, Inc., Chicago, Illinois.)

j. Negative energy balance.

(1) Excessive weight loss due to negative energy balance is a potential problem during deployment to high altitude regions. Weight loss was the sixth most common occurrence in Soldiers deployed to Afghanistan. Excessive weight loss can have detrimental effects on combat performance. Energy requirements for high altitude operations are increased above sea-level requirements. The altitude, cold temperatures, and performance of physical activities over rugged terrain combine to increase energy expenditures to as much as 4,500 kilocalorie (kcal) per day. Negative energy balance is the result of increased energy expenditure and decreased

food intake due to anorexia and behavioral phenomenon at high altitude. Anorexia can be the result of AMS and hypohydration. Hypoxia-induced malaise effect on judgment and reasoning can limit intake of food and fluid.

(2) Medical providers need to be prepared to treat personnel with excessive weight loss as well as advise their commanders on proper nutrition and caloric requirements to prevent such incidents at high altitude. Prevention of weight loss is not entirely possible but encouraging units to eat small, frequent, meals rather than large, infrequent meals will help. At approximately 1,300 kcal per ration, the current Meal, Ready to Eat does not supply adequate energy to sustain combat operations. The First Strike Ration™ may be a better option at 2,900 kcal per ration. Most healthy Soldiers tolerate the weight loss fairly well and recover the weight when they redeploy to low altitude. (First Strike Ration® is a registered trademark of the Department of the Army.)

k. Constipation and hemorrhoids. Constipation and acute exacerbation of hemorrhoids are common during high altitude deployments due to changes in dietary consumption patterns, reduced water intake and voluntary delay of defecation to avoid cold or unsheltered areas. Both conditions can adversely affect physical performance as well as the mood of Soldiers. Normal bowel movements can usually be maintained with an adequate fluid intake and the inclusion of fruits or other sources of fiber in the diet. Soldiers with preexisting hemorrhoids should have them medically evaluated and, if necessary, treated to prevent exacerbation during deployment to high altitude areas. Constipation and hemorrhoids occurring during high altitude deployment can be treated according to standard clinical guidelines including hydration, dietary manipulations, mineral oil (1 tablespoon twice a day) for lubrication, mild anesthetics, such as dibucaine, hemorrhoidal suppositories, or hydrocortisone ointment. Medical personnel should insure that sufficient supplies of these materials are available during deployment.

6–4. Preexisting medical conditions
  a. Introduction.
  (1) A number of acute and chronic medical conditions that may be present in Soldiers before deployment to high altitude can interact with hypobaric hypoxia and either worsen the underlying condition itself or aggravate the hypoxia making the Soldier more susceptible to altitude illness. Medications that Soldiers may be taking during deployment to treat preexisting medical conditions may also increase the risk of altitude illness (see appendix E for dosing recommendations for primary altitude illness medications and contraindications). Chronic conditions or medications that affect the cardiovascular and/or respiratory systems are obvious risks at high altitude and may be contraindicated. Examples include chronic obstructive pulmonary disease, unstable angina, poorly controlled arrhythmia, congestive heart failure, congenital and acquired valvular heart disease, unrevascularized coronary artery disease, pulmonary hypertension, anemia, high-risk pregnancy, and medications that depress respiration. Any blood-clotting abnormality as evidenced by a history of stroke or abnormal laboratory values carries a greatly increased risk of altitude-related embolic events. Both sleep apnea and obesity can exaggerate hypoxemia. Temporary or acute medical conditions which can increase the health risk of Soldiers deployed to high mountain environments include infections (especially upper and lower respiratory tract infections) and high-risk pregnancies.

(2) Many chronic medical conditions that can cause problems at high altitude will normally disqualify Soldiers from active duty (AR 40–501) or prevent them from being deployed. However, given the aging military population as well as increased vigilance in retaining highly qualified Soldiers, medical officers should be aware of conditions in Soldiers that might increase their health risks when deployed to high altitude. Predeployment medical screening should be conducted to identify individuals with preexisting acute or chronic medical problems. If a significant condition is discovered during predeployment screening, that Soldier should be evaluated for a temporary or permanent physical profile to limit their altitude exposure. Most individuals with conditions such as hypertension, coronary artery disease, diabetes, mild to moderate chronic obstructive pulmonary disease, asthma, migraine, sleep-disordered breathing, or low-risk pregnancy tolerate altitude but might require monitoring and careful review of existing medications and potential for adverse interactions (see appendix E).

   b. *Hematologic conditions.*

   (1) Sickle cell trait is a chronic condition that does not normally disqualify a Soldier from active duty. However, altitude exposure greatly increases the risk of sickle crisis with splenic sequestration and infarction during altitude exposure. The risk for this complication may be higher in non-black Soldiers with sickle trait than it is in black Soldiers with the trait. The differential diagnosis of left upper quadrant pain at altitude (even as low as 1,500 m) should include splenic infarction. All Soldiers with sickle cell trait should be evaluated carefully prior to high altitude deployment. Those with a high degree of sickling at low oxygen tensions should be considered for a physical profile to limit altitude exposure.

   (2) Anemia, where oxygen-carrying capacity is reduced, should be treated prior to ascent. Given the central role of hemoglobin in oxygen transport, a low hemoglobin level might be expected to affect tolerance to high altitude. Premenopausal women may have inadequate iron stores to effectively support increased erythropoiesis at altitude and might benefit from iron therapy before or during a deployment to altitude. Soldiers with recurrent clotting or bleeding problems should not go to altitude.

   c. *Respiratory conditions.*

   (1) Transfer of oxygen from air to blood is the first stage of oxygen transport and the function of the respiratory system. Components of this system include control of ventilation, pulmonary mechanics, matching of ventilation and perfusion in the lung, and gas exchange across the capillary membrane. Medical conditions affecting any of these factors may impair oxygenation, especially at high altitude, where adjustments in the respiratory system are crucial for well-being.

   (2) Disorders of ventilatory control include carotid body ablation and sleep-disordered breathing and apnea. Carotid body responsiveness to hypoxia is generally considered necessary for optimal acclimatization to altitude. Sleep-disordered breathing and apnea might also increase nocturnal hypoxemia at high altitude. Chronic obstructive pulmonary disease, such as chronic bronchitis and emphysema, is the most common cause of impaired oxygen transport, and thus would be expected to impact those traveling to high altitude. Smoking is another factor that would impair oxygen transport and should be discouraged at high altitude. Although airflow obstruction, such as during an asthmatic attack, would be expected to produce more hyoxemia at

altitude than at sea level, neither data nor anecdotal reports validate this possibility. Limited data suggest that high altitude appears not to exacerbate asthma and actually improves allergic asthma due to decreased allergens and pollution.

  d. *Cardiovascular conditions.*

  (1) Preexisting arterial hypertension may exacerbate the blood pressure response to altitude. Some individuals develop severe hypertension at altitude, but the magnitude of the blood pressure response may depend on the hypoxic stress. The medications used to control hypertension, such as loop diuretics, should be carefully evaluated before administering altitude illness medications to such individuals. Administering a mild diuretic (acetazolamide) on top of another diuretic may be contraindicated. A theoretical basis for exacerbation of coronary artery disease at high altitude exists. Cardiac work is slightly increased at altitude, and the usual compensatory increase in coronary blood flow may not be attained in those with coronary artery disease. Small increases in heart rate and blood pressure on initial ascent to altitude may cause angina or induce angina in those with coronary artery disease.

  (2) Cold exposure may provoke myocardial ischemia at high altitude, as it is known to do at low altitude. No one with known coronary artery disease or significant risk factors for coronary artery disease should undertake unaccustomed exercise at high altitude.

  (a) Soldiers with preexisting troublesome or high-grade arrhythmia have not been evaluated systematically at high altitude, and anecdotal reports of exacerbation of supraventricular tachycardia or other common arrhythmias are largely word of mouth. Although the hypoxemia of moderate altitude does not depress myocardial contractility, the tendency toward fluid retention in some at altitude, especially with AMS, could aggravate heart failure. The hypoxia of high altitude elevates pulmonary arterial pressure and resistance. As a result, congenital heart disease conditions, such as atrial and ventricular septal defects, patent ductus arteriosus, and partially corrected tetralogy of Fallot, might have increased right-to-left shunting at high altitude. This may exacerbate desaturation in these Soldiers.

  (b) In addition to congenital cardiac defects, any illness resulting in pulmonary hypertension is contraindicated with high altitude exposure. Hypoxic pulmonary vasoconstriction will most likely exaggerate preexisting pulmonary hypertension. Given the prominent role of pulmonary hypertension in the pathophysiology of HAPE, any such illness may predispose an individual to HAPE.

  e. *Neurological conditions.* There is anecdotal evidence that altitude tends to trigger migraine attacks which can be severe. The headache of AMS and that of migraine can be nearly indistinguishable, and this presents obvious problems. Stroke, TIA and cerebrovascular disorders may be increased at high altitude. Because of the significant cerebral vasodilation on ascent to high altitude, persons with cerebrovascular structural abnormalities, such as aneurysm, or recent traumatic brain injury may be at risk for an untoward event. Acute, severe hypoxia may cause a seizure. In persons with seizure disorders, exacerbation possibly due to altitude has been anecdotally observed.

  f. *Metabolic conditions.* Glucose tolerance is normal at altitude when energy expenditure and food intake balance one another. Exercise at altitude may improve sugar intake and, for well-controlled diabetics, there appears to be no contraindication to high altitude exposure. Ready access to glucose in the form of sugar or chocolate is necessary, and intravenous glucose should be available for emergencies as hypoglycemia can be produced very rapidly by intense sustained activity. Hypothermia can produce hypoglycemia, and exhausted diabetic Soldiers are at considerable risk.

g. *Ophthalmological conditions.* The parts of the eye most affected by altitude are the cornea and the retina. Hypoxia disturbs the homeostasis of corneal fluid balance, and the cornea diffusely swells especially after lid closure during sleep. Since the swelling is uniform, there is no change in corneal curvature and no visual abnormality occurs. Persons who have had radial keratotomy (RK) for refraction correction, however, no longer have structurally normal corneas. On ascent to altitude, the swelling of the hypoxic cornea is not uniform in these cases, and significant visual changes may occur and cause visual blurring. In contrast, photorefractive keratectomy (PRK) is a laser technique that shaves the anterior cornea uniformly, and no changes in vision occur at high altitude in these individuals. Contact lenses may be used successfully at high altitude, but use at altitude entails several considerations beyond those encountered in normal use. Overnight use of extended-wear contact lenses is not recommended because of associated increased rate of microbial keratitis. Contact lens wearers should always have backup glasses available for use and carry both fluoroquinolone and rewetting drops.

h. *Psychiatric conditions.* At very high altitudes, individuals can experience hostile behavior changes, with thoughts of paranoia, depression, anxiety and obsessive-compulsiveness predominating. Those at intermediate altitudes do not experience any behavior changes consistent with increased aggressiveness. Feelings of diminished vigor, weariness, and increased sleepiness are commonly experienced at intermediate altitudes. There are three types of anxiety-related disorders that have been related to altitude exposure: limited-symptom panic attacks induced by nocturnal periodic breathing, excessive health-related anxiety, and excessive emotionality. Individuals with preexisting psychiatric conditions should be carefully evaluated before deployment to high altitude.

i. *Gastrointestinal conditions.* Gastrointestinal bleeding is not uncommon at altitude. Clearly, patients with known peptic ulcers should not go to altitude unless the disease is well-controlled. Those with inflammatory disorders of the bowel, such as Crohn's disease or ulcerative colitis, should also not go to altitude. Soldiers with hernias should have them repaired before going to altitude.

j. *Pregnancy.* Pregnant women will not be deployed to high altitude in the military. However, pregnant women may be stationed at moderate altitude. Low-risk pregnancy should not be affected by moderate altitude, but high-risk pregnancy may be contraindicated.

k. *Pharmacologically active substances.*

(1) Substances with pharmacologic activity can interact with effects of hypobaric hypoxia, environmental/mission factors and preexisting medical conditions to cause medical problems at high altitude. There are several possible sources of pharmacologically active substances. Prescription drugs are an obvious source, and medical officers not only must take into account the effects of drugs they themselves may prescribe during altitude deployment, but also must be aware of any drugs, such as blood pressure medication, that a Soldier may take chronically. Soldiers often bring nonprescription ("over-the-counter") medications with them during deployment, and medical personnel may not be aware of these unless they ask individual

Soldiers. Illicit drugs are a potential source of pharmacologically active substances that should not be ignored. Other common sources of pharmacologically active substances are caffeine, tobacco, and alcoholic beverages.

(2) Because hypobaric hypoxia is ubiquitous at high altitude, any substance that interferes with oxygen delivery is a significant threat. Examples include sedatives, sleeping aids, tranquilizers, and other medications that depress respiration. Tobacco smoke interferes with oxygen delivery by reduction of blood oxygen-carrying capacity through increased carboxyhemoglobin levels. Oxygen-carrying capacity can be reduced by as much as 5 to 10 percent by tobacco smoke. Additionally, the irritant effect of tobacco smoke may produce a narrowing of small airways, interfering with optimal air movement. The combination can effectively raise the "physiological altitude" as much as several hundred meters.

(3) Substances with significant diuretic properties, such as alcoholic beverages, caffeine, and diuretic medications, can be a problem at high altitude where Soldiers have decreased plasma volume and are often dehydrated due to decreased fluid intake and fluid losses from altitude illness. Acetazolmide, used to both prevent and treat AMS, is a fairly weak diuretic but when used in combination with other diuretics may be a problem. Substances which cause significant peripheral vasodilation are also a theoretical hazard at high altitude due to altitude-associated decreases in plasma volume. Additionally, hypoxia-induced peripheral vasodilation accelerates heat loss and makes Soldiers more vulnerable to hypothermia and frostbite. Peripheral vasodilation is a well-known effect of alcohol. Substances which cause peripheral vasoconstriction also increase the risk of cold injury. Peripheral vasoconstriction caused by tobacco products increases the risk for freezing cold injuries.

(4) Medications and other substances that alter mental status interact with hypoxia-induced decrements in cerebral function to greatly increase the chance of errors in judgment and accidents. Alcohol impairs judgment and perception and promotes psychomotor dysfunction. Alcohol also depresses respiration, causes hypoglycemia, and induces an undesirable diuresis. Unlike alcohol, caffeine from coffee and tea improves physical and mental performance. It also causes diuresis and, therefore, should be consumed in moderation. Caffeine users must maintain adequate hydration.

APPENDIX A

REFERENCES

Section I
Required Publications
Except as noted below, Army regulations are available online from the U.S. Army Publishing Directorate Web site: http://www.apd.army.mil. Field manuals are available online from the General Dennis J. Reimer Training and Doctrine Digital Library Web site: http://www.train.army.mil. Technical bulletins, medical are available online from the U.S. Army Public Health Command (Provisional) (USAPHC (Prov)), formerly known as U.S. Army Center for Health Promotion and Preventive Medicine (USACHPPM), Web site: http://phc.amedd.army.mil. U.S. Army Research Institute of Environmental Medicine (USARIEM) publications are available online from the USARIEM Web site: http://www.usariem.army.mil/Pages/downloads.htm. Chapters from the *Textbooks of Military Medicine: Medical Aspects of Harsh Environments Volume 2* are available online from the Office of The Surgeon General, Borden Institute Web site: http://www.bordeninstitute.army.mil/published_volumes/harshEnv2/harshEnv2.html.)

AR 40–501
Standards of Medical Fitness (Cited in para 2-4*b*, and 6–4*a*(2).)

FM 5–19
Composite Risk Management (Cited in para 3–1*c*.) (Available at https://rdl.train.army.mil/soldierPortal/atia/adlsc/view/public/23137-1/FM/5-19/FM5_19.PDF.)

TB MED 507/AFPAM 48–152(I)
Heat Stress Control and Heat Casualty Management (Cited in paras 3–5*a*(1), 6–3*d*(2), and 6–3*i*(2).)

TB MED 508
Prevention and Management of Cold-Weather Injuries (Cited in para 6–3*c*(2).)

Section II
Related Publications
A related publication is a source of additional information. The user does not have to read it to understand this publication.

AR 40–5
Preventive Medicine

TB MED 505

AR 40–400
Patient Administration

FM 3–97.6
Mountain Operations

FM 3–97.61
Military Mountaineering

FM 4–02.17
Preventive Medicine Services

FM 4–25.12
Unit Field Sanitation Team

FM 8–55
Planning for Health Service Support

TB MED 288
Medical Problems of Man at High Terrestrial Elevations

USARIEM Technical Note TN04–05
Altitude Acclimatization Guide

USARIEM Technical Note TN94–2
Medical Problems in High Mountain Environments: A Handbook for Medical Officers

USARIEM Technical Report T3/85
Relationship between the Army Two-Mile Run Test and Maximal Oxygen Uptake. (Available at http://handle.dtic.mil/100.2/ADA153914.)

U.S. Government Printing Office
U.S. Standard Atmosphere, 1962 (Available at http://handle.dtic.mil/100.2/AD659893.)

International Civil Aviation Organization
Manual of ICAO Standard Atmosphere (extended to 80 kilometres (262,500 feet) (Available at http://www.icao.int.)

Marine Corps Center for Lessons Learned (MCCLL) January 2007 Newsletter
Medical Support of Operations in a High Altitude, Mountainous Environment: Quick Look Report (Available at http://www.mccll.usmc.mil.)

Section III
Prescribed Forms
This section contains no entries.

Section IV
Referenced Forms
This section contains no entries.

Section V
Selected Bibliography

Banderet, L.E., and B. Shukitt-Hale. 2002. Cognitive performance, mood, and neurological status at high terrestrial elevations. In *Textbooks of Military Medicine: Medical Aspects of Harsh Environments Volume 2*, ed. D.E. Lounsbury, R.F. Bellamy, and R. Zajtchuk, 725–759. Washington, DC: Office of The Surgeon General, Borden Institute.

Fulco, C.S., and A. Cymerman. 1988. Human performance and acute hypoxia. In *Human Performance Physiology and Environmental Medicine at Terrestrial Extremes*, ed. K.B. Pandolf, M.N. Sawka, and R.R. Gonzalez, 467–495. Indianapolis: Benchmark Press, Inc. (Available at http://handle.dtic.mil/100.2/ADA192604.)

Fulco, C.S., and A. Cymerman. 2002. Physical performance at varying terrestrial altitudes. In *Textbooks of Military Medicine: Medical Aspects of Harsh Environments Volume 2*, ed. D.E. Lounsbury, R.F. Bellamy, and R. Zajtchuk, 689–724. Washington, D.C.: Office of The Surgeon General, Borden Institute.

Fulco, C.S., K.W. Kambis, A.L. Friedlander, P.B. Rock, S.R. Muza, and A. Cymerman. 2005. Carbohydrate supplementation improves time-trial cycle performance during energy deficit at 4,300-m altitude. *J Appl Physiol* 99(3): 867–876.

Fulco, C.S., P.B. Rock, and A. Cymerman. 1998. Maximal and submaximal exercise performance at altitude. *Aviat Space Environ Med* 69(8): 793–801.

Gallagher, S.A., and P.H. Hackett. 2004. High-altitude illness. *Emerg Med Clin North Am* 22(2): 329–355, viii.

Luks, A.M. 2008. Which medicines are safe and effective for improving sleep at high altitude? *High Alt Med Biol* 9(3): 195–198.

Muza, S.R. 2007. Military applications of hypoxic training for high-altitude operations. *Med Sci Sports Exerc* 39(9): 1625–1631.

Roach, J.M., and R.B. Schoene. 2002. High-altitude pulmonary edema. In *Textbooks of Military Medicine: Medical Aspects of Harsh Environments Volume 2*, ed. D.E. Lounsbury, R.F. Bellamy, and R. Zajtchuk, 789–814. Washington, D.C.: Office of The Surgeon General, Borden Institute.

Roach, R., J. Stepanek, and P. Hackett. 2002. Acute mountain sickness and high-altitude cerebral edema. In *Textbooks of Military Medicine: Medical Aspects of Harsh Environments Volume 2*, ed. D.E. Lounsbury, R.F. Bellamy, and R. Zajtchuk, 760–788. Washington, D.C.: Office of The Surgeon General, Borden Institute.

Rock, P.B. and E.J. Iwanyk. 2002. Military medical operations in mountain environments. In *Textbooks of Military Medicine: Medical Aspects of Harsh Environments Volume 2*, ed. D.E. Lounsbury, R.F. Bellamy, and R. Zajtchuk, 854–869. Washington, D.C.: Office of The Surgeon General, Borden Institute.

Rock, P.B., and T.H. Mader. 2002. Additional medical problems in mountain environments. In *Textbooks of Military Medicine: Medical Aspects of Harsh Environments Volume 2*, ed. D.E. Lounsbury, R.F. Bellamy, and R. Zajtchuk, 815–853. Washington, D.C.: Office of The Surgeon General, Borden Institute.

Wilderness Medical Society. 2001. *Wilderness Medical Society Practice Guidelines for Wilderness Emergency Care*, 2d ed, 43. Guilford, Connecticut: The Globe Pequot Press.

Young, A.J., and J.T. Reeves. 2002. Human adaptation to high terrestrial altitude. In *Textbooks of Military Medicine: Medical Aspects of Harsh Environments Volume 2*, ed. D.E. Lounsbury, R.F. Bellamy, and R. Zajtchuk, 644–688. Washington, D.C.: Office of The Surgeon General, Borden Institute.

Young, A.J., and P.M. Young. 1988. Human acclimatization to high terrestrial altitude. In *Human Performance Physiology and Environmental Medicine at Terrestrial Extremes*, ed. K.B. Pandolf, M.N. Sawka, and R.R. Gonzalez, 497–543. Indianapolis: Benchmark Press, Inc.

APPENDIX B

COUNTRIES AND ELEVATIONS

Table B–1
Highest elevation and geographical point of countries within each of the continents

Rank	Nation	Highest Elevation (m)	Highest Geographical Point
North America			
1	United States	6,194	Mount McKinley
2	Canada	5,959	Mount Logan
3	Mexico	5,700	Volcan Pico de Orizaba
4	Greenland	3,700	Gunnbjorn
5	Dominican Republic	3,175	Pico Duarte
6	Haiti	2,680	Chaine de la Selle
7	Jamaica	2,256	Blue Mountain Peak
8	Cuba	2,005	Pico Turquino
9	Dominica	1,447	Morne Diablatins
10	Puerto Rico	1,339	Cerro de Punta
11	Saint Vincent & the Grenadines	1,234	La Soufriere
South America			
1	Argentina	6,960	Cerro Aconcagua
2	Chile	6,880	Nevado Ojos del Salado
3	Peru	6,768	Nevado Huascaran
4	Bolivia	6,542	Nevado Sajama
5	Ecuador	6,267	Chimborazo
6	Colombia	5,881	Pico Cristobal Colon & Pico Simon Bolivar
7	Venezuela	5,007	Pico Bolivar (La Columna)
8	Guatemala	4,211	Volcan Tajumulco
9	Costa Rica	3,810	Cerro Chirripo
10	Panama	3,475	Volcan Baru
11	Brazil	3,014	Pico da Neblina
12	South Georgia & the South Sandwich Islands	2,934	Mount Paget (South Georgia)
13	Honduras	2,870	Cerro Las Minas
14	Guyana	2,835	Mount Roraima
15	El Salvador	2,730	Cerro El Pital
16	Nicaragua	2,438	Mogoton
17	Suriname	1,230	Juliana Top

Table B–1
Highest elevation and geographical point of countries within each of the continents
(continued)

Rank	Nation	Highest Elevation (m)	Highest Geographical Point
Europe			
1	Turkey	5,166	Mount Ararat
2	France	4,807	Mont Blanc
3	Italy	4,748	Mont Blanc (Monte Bianco) de Courmayeur
4	Switzerland	4,634	Dufourspitze
5	Austria	3,798	Grossglockner
6	Spain	3,718	Pico de Teide (Tenerife) on Canary Islands
7	Germany	2,963	Zugspitze
8	Andorra	2,946	Coma Pedrosa
9	Bulgaria	2,925	Musala
10	Greece	2,917	Mount Olympus
11	Slovenia	2,864	Triglav
12	Macedonia & Albania	2,764	Golem Korab (Maja e Korabit)
13	Serbia	2,656	Daravica
14	Slovakia	2,655	Gerlachovsky Stit
15	Liechtenstein	2,599	Vorder-Grauspitz
16	Romania	2,544	Moldoveanu
17	Montenegro	2,522	Bobotov Kuk
18	Poland	2,499	Rysy
19	Norway	2,469	Galdhopiggen
20	Bosnia and Herzegovina	2,386	Maglic
21	Portugal	2,351	Ponta do Pico (Pico or Pico Alto) on Ilha do Pico in the Azores
22	Jan Mayen	2,277	Haakon VII Toppen/Beerenberg
23	Sweden	2,111	Kebnekaise
24	Iceland	2,110	Hvannadalshnukur (at Vatnajokull Glacier)
25	Ukraine	2,061	Hora Hoverla
26	Croatia	1,830	Dinara
27	Svalbard	1,717	Newtontoppen
28	Czech Republic	1,602	Snezka
29	United Kingdom	1,343	Ben Nevis
30	Finland	1,328	Haltiatunturi

Table B–1
Highest elevation and geographical point of countries within each of the continents (continued)

Rank	Nation	Highest Elevation (m)	Highest Geographical Point
		Africa	
1	Tanzania	5,895	Kilimanjaro
2	Kenya	5,199	Mount Kenya
3	Uganda & Democratic Republic of the Congo	5,110	Margherita Peak on Mount Stanley
4	Ethiopia	4,620	Ras Dejen
5	Rwanda	4,519	Volcan Karisimbi
6	Morocco	4,165	Jebel Toubkal
7	Cameron	4,095	Fako (on Mount Cameroon)
8	Lesotho	3,482	Thabana Ntlenyana
9	Chad	3,415	Emi Koussi
10	South Africa	3,408	Njesuthi
11	Sudan	3,187	Kinyeti
12	Eritrea	3,018	Soira
13	Equatorial Guinea	3,008	Pico Basile
14	Algeria	3,003	Tahat
15	Malawi	3,002	Sapitwa (Mount Mlanje)
16	Madagascar	2,876	Maromokotro
17	Burundi	2,670	Heha
18	Egypt	2,629	Mount Catherine
19	Angola	2,620	Morro de Moco
20	Konigstein	2,606	Konigstein
21	Zimbabwe	2,592	Inyangani
22	Mozambique	2,436	Monte Binga
23	Nigeria	2,419	Chappal Waddi
24	Somalia	2,416	Shimbiris
25	Comoros	2,360	Le Kartala
26	Zambia	2,301	Unnamed Location in Mafinga Hills
27	Libya	2,267	Bikku Bitti
28	Saint Helena	2,062	Queen Mary's Peak on Tristan da Cunha
29	Djibouti	2,028	Moussa Ali
30	Sao Tome and Principe	2,024	Pico de Sao Tome
31	Niger	2,022	Mont Bagzane
32	Sierra Leone	1,948	Loma Mansa (Bintimani)
33	Swaziland	1,862	Emlembe
34	Guinea & Cote d'Ivoire	1,752	Mont Nimba

Table B–1
Highest elevation and geographical point of countries within each of the continents
(continued)

Rank	Nation	Highest Elevation (m)	Highest Geographical Point
Africa (continued)			
35	Gabon	1,575	Mont Iboundji
36	Tunisia	1,544	Jebel ech Chambi
37	Botswana	1,489	Tsodilo Hills
38	Central African Republic	1,420	Mont Ngaoui
39	Liberia	1,380	Mount Wuteve
Asia			
1	Nepal & China	8,850	Mount Everest
2	Pakistan	8,611	K2 (Mount Godwin-Austen)
3	India	8,598	Kanchenjunga
4	Bhutan	7,553	Kula Kangri
5	Tajikistan	7,495	Qullai Ismoili Somoni
6	Afghanistan	7,485	Nowshak
7	Kyrgyztan	7,439	Jengish Chokusu (Pik Pobedy)
8	Kazakhstan	6,995	Khan Tangiri Shyngy (Pik Khan-Tengri)
9	Burma	5,881	Hkakabo Razi
10	Iran	5,671	Kuh-e Damavand
11	Russia	5,633	Gora El'brus
12	Georgia	5,201	Mt'a Shkhara
13	Indonesia	5,030	Puncak Jaya
14	Azerbaijan	4,485	Bazarduzu Dagi
15	Mongolia	4,374	Nayramadlin Orgil (Huyten Orgil)
16	Uzbekistan	4,301	Adelunga Toghi
17	Malaysia	4,100	Gunung Kinabalu
18	Armenia	4,090	Aragats Lerrnagagat'
19	Taiwan	3,952	Yu Shan
20	Japan	3,776	Mount Fuji
21	Yemen	3,760	Jabal an Nabi Shu'ayb
22	Iraq	3,611	Unnamed Peak
23	Vietnam	3,144	Fan Si Pan
24	Turkmenistan	3,139	Gora Ayribaba
25	Saudi Arabia	3,133	Jabal Sawda'
26	Lebanon	3,088	Qurnat as Sawda'
27	Oman	2,980	Jabal Shams
28	East Timor	2,963	Foho Tatamailau

Table B–1
Highest elevation and geographical point of countries within each of the continents (continued)

Rank	Nation	Highest Elevation (m)	Highest Geographical Point
Asia (continued)			
29	Philippines	2,954	Mount Apo
30	Laos	2,817	Phou Bia
31	Syria	2,814	Mount Hermon
32	Heard Island & McDonald Islands	2,745	Mawson Peak, on Big Ben
33	North Korea	2,744	Paektu-san
34	Thailand	2,576	Doi Inthanon
35	Sri Lanka	2,524	Pidurutalagala
36	Cyprus	1,951	Mount Olympus
37	South Korea	1,950	Halla-san
38	Brunei	1,850	Bukit Pagon
39	Cambodia	1,810	Phnum Aoral
40	Jordan	1,734	Jabal Ram
41	United Arab Emirates	1,527	Jabal Yibir
42	Bangladesh	1,230	Keokradong
43	Israel	1,208	Har Meron
Oceania			
1	Papua New Guinea	4,509	Mount Wilhelm
2	New Zealand	3,754	Aoraki-Mount Cook
3	Solomon Islands	2,447	Mount Makarakomburu
4	French Polynesia	2,241	Mont Orohena
5	Australia	2,229	Mount Kosciuszko
6	Vanuatu	1,877	Tabwemasana
7	Samoa	1,857	Mauga Silisili (Savaii)
8	New Caledonia	1,628	Mont Panie
9	Fiji	1,324	Tomanivi
Antarctica			
1	Antarctica	4,897	Vinson Massif
2	French Southern & Antarctic Lands	1,850	Mont Ross on Iles Kerguelen

This page intentionally left blank

APPENDIX C

MAXIMAL OXYGEN UPTAKE AND TWO-MILE RUN TIME

Table C-1
Estimating maximal oxygen uptake for men and women using two-mile run time

Two-Mile Time (min)	Men (mL/kg/min)	Women (mL/kg/min)
10	66	55
11	63	53
12	60	52
13	56	50
14	53	48
15	49	46
16	46	45
17	43	43
18	39	41
19	36	39
20	33	38
21	29	36
22	26	34
23	23	32
24		30
25		29
26		27
27		25
28		23

Legend:
mL/kg/min = milliliters of oxygen consumed for each kilogram of body weight per minute.

This page intentionally left blank

APPENDIX D

FIRST AID FOR HIGH ALTITUDE PROBLEMS

Table D–1
Summary of treatments for some common altitude-related problems

Summary	Diagnosis	Treatment
Headache only	High altitude headache	Ibuprofen, acetaminophen, aspirin
Headache and insomnia, fatigue, dizziness, anorexia, or nausea	Acute mountain sickness	Descent; stop, rest and acclimatize; acetazolamide (250 mg b.i.d.); prochlorperazine (10 mg three times daily (t.i.d.)) for nausea.
Gait ataxia, altered mental status, severe lassitude	High altitude cerebral edema	Immediate descent, supplementary oxygen (4–6 L/min), hyperbaric bag treatment, dexamethasone (8 mg initially, then 4 mg every 6 hrs).
Decreased exercise performance, dry cough, dyspnea at rest, wheezing, tachypnea, tachycardia, blood-tinged sputum	High altitude pulmonary edema	Immediate descent; supplementary oxygen (2–4 L/min); hyperbaric bag treatment, nifedipine (10 mg initially, then 30 mg extended release every 12 to 24 hrs).
Persistent dry cough	High altitude pharyngitis/bronchitis	Mild cough suppressant, throat lozenges, steam inhalation, breathable silk balaclava.
Body weight gain, swelling of face and extremities	Altitude-induced peripheral edema	Acetazolamide, 250 mg t.i.d. for 1 day; salt restriction.
Body weight loss, difficulty sleeping, impaired judgment	Chronic fatigue (energy depletion)	Proper diet, rest, and rehydration. Eat several small meals per day.
Tired and weak, dry throat, dark urine, rapid heartbeat, headache, dizziness	Dehydration	Rest and rehydration. Severe cases require intravenous rehydration. Oral electrolyte solution helpful.
Abdominal pain, weakness and nausea, frequent diarrhea, loss of appetite	Parasitical/bacterial illness (that is, traveler's diarrhea)	Norfloxacin 400 mg b.i.d. for 3 days (bacterial); metronidazole 500 mg t.i.d. for 7 days (viral).
Insomnia	Altitude-related sleep problems	Acetazolamide, 250 mg t.i.d.
Poor vision, dark spots	High altitude retinal hemorrhage or snow blindness	Descent.
Pain, swelling in limb, chest pain, dyspnea, hypoxemia, neurological deficiency	Thromboembolic event	Low-dose subcutaneous heparin (5,000 units every 8–12 hrs).

This page intentionally left blank

APPENDIX E

MEDICAL THERAPY FOR HIGH ALTITUDE ILLNESS AND CONTRAINDICATIONS

Table E-1
Medical treatments for altitude illnesses and other altitude-related problems

Agent	Indications	Prevention Dose	Treatment Dose	Adverse Effects	Comments	Contraindications
Oxygen	All high altitude illnesses		2–4 L/min by cannula or mask initially, then titrate dose until SaO$_2$ >90%.		Lifesaving for HAPE; improves headache within minutes for AMS.	
Portable hyperbaric chamber	All high altitude illnesses		Depends on model; 2–4 psi for a minimum of 2 hrs; continue as long as necessary.	Potential rebound effect after removal.	Effects equivalent to the administration of low-flow oxygen; can be lifesaving; for maximal effect, add supplemental oxygen.	May provoke anxiety. Use caution in Soldiers with previous anxiety disorders.
Acetazolamide	AMS Sleep disturbances	125 to 250 mg orally twice daily, or one 500 mg extended release 24 hrs prior to ascent and first 48 hrs at high altitude	250 mg orally twice daily or one 500 mg extended-release capsule until symptoms resolve.	Parasthesias; alters taste of carbonated beverages; polyuria.	Sulfoamide reactions possible.	Hepatic insufficiency; avoid in Soldiers using long-term aspirin or with ventilatory limitation (forced expiratory volume (FEV) <25% predicted), sulfa allergy.
Dexamethasone	AMS	4 mg every 6 to 8 hrs orally 24 hrs prior to ascent	4 mg every 6 to 8 hrs orally, intravenously, or intramuscularly.	Mood changes, hyperglycemia, dyspepsia, rebound effect on withdrawal; hypertension; sodium and water retention; prolonged wound healing; gastrointestinal (GI) bleeding.	Can be lifesaving for AMS or HACE; effects evident in 2–8 hrs; no effect on acclimatization; may also prevent HAPE.	Expect elevated blood glucose values in diabetics. Avoid in Soldiers with peptic ulcer disease or upper-GI bleeding. Caution in Soldiers at risk for amebiasis or strongyloidiasis. Avoid with systemic fungal infections.
	HACE		8 mg initially, then 4 mg every 6 hrs orally, intravenously, or intramuscularly.			

Table E–1
Medical treatments for altitude illnesses and other altitude-related problems **(continued)**

Agent	Indications	Prevention Dose	Treatment Dose	Adverse Effects	Comments	Contraindications
Furosemide	AMS or HACE		80 mg orally every 12 hrs for a total of 2 doses.	Hypovolemia; dry mouth; hypotension; hypokalemia.	Currently out of favor.	Anuria, hypovolemia, state of electrolyte depletion.
Nifedipine	HAPE	30 mg of extended release formulation orally every 12–24 hrs	10 mg orally initially, then 30 mg of extended-release formulation orally every 12–24 hrs.	Reflex tachycardia; increased risk of gastroesophageal reflux.	No value in AMS or HACE.	Pregnancy and lactation, severe hypotension, hepatic insufficiency. Caution in Soldiers at risk for GI bleeding. Caution when using in Soldiers receiving other antihypertensive medications. Avoid grapefruit juice and calcium supplements and NSAIDs.
Tadalafil	HAPE	10 mg orally twice a day	Unknown	Flushing, headache, dyspepsia, visual disturbance, rhinitis, gastroesophageal reflux.	Preventive measure only. May exacerbate AMS.	Avoid concurrent use of nitrates and α-blockers. Dose adjustments necessary in renal and hepatic disease.
Sildenafil	HAPE	50 mg every 8 hrs	Unknown	Flushing; headache; dyspepsia; visual disturbance; GI reflux.	Preventive measure only. May exacerbate AMS.	Avoid concurrent use of nitrates and α-blockers. Dose adjustments necessary in renal and hepatic insufficiency.
Salmeterol	HAPE	125 μg inhaled twice daily	Unknown	Sinus headache, nausea, throat irritation, sleep disturbance, parasethesia.	Preventive measure only.	Caution in Soldiers receiving chloroquine for malaria prophylaxis. Caution in Soldiers receiving monoamine oxidase inhibitors and tricyclic antidepressants. Caution in Soldiers with predisposition toward hypokalemia. Avoid concurrent use of ß-blockers. Avoid in hepatic insufficiency.
Aspirin	AMS headache	325 mg orally every 4 hrs beginning 2 hrs before ascent for a total of 3 doses		Dyspepsia, GI bleeding, dizziness, confusion, nausea, heartburn.	Preventive measure only.	History of GI insufficiency; pregnancy; hemophilia or other bleeding disorders.
Acetaminophen	AMS headache		325 to 1,000 mg every 4 hrs, not to exceed 4,000 mg daily.		Acetaminophen as effective as ibuprofen in relieving headache.	Overdose can result in liver toxicity, failure or even death. Avoid in Soldiers with liver and kidney disease.
Ibuprofen	AMS headache		400–600 mg orally every 4–6 hrs, not to exceed 3,200 mg daily.	Dyspepsia, GI bleeding, nausea, heartburn, dizziness, rash.	Treatment only.	Do not initiate treatment in dehydrated Soldiers.

Table E–1
Medical treatments for altitude illnesses and other altitude-related problems (continued)

Agent	Indications	Prevention Dose	Treatment Dose	Adverse Effects	Comments	Contraindications
Prochlorperazine	Nausea/ vomiting		10 mg orally or intramuscularly every 6–8 hrs.	Extrapyramidal reactions; may cause dizziness, drowsiness or blurred vision.	Use diphenhydramine intramuscularly for extrapyramidal reactions.	Avoid prolonged exposure to sunlight. Caution in use with bone marrow disease, glaucoma, seizure, Parkinson's disease, kidney disease, liver disease, and pregnancy.
Promethazine	Nausea/ vomiting		25–50 mg orally, intramuscularly or rectally every 6 hrs.	Extrapyramidal reactions; cause sedation.	Use diphenhydramine intramuscularly for extrapyramidal reactions.	Avoid prolonged exposure to sunlight. Caution in use with bone marrow disease, glaucoma, seizure, Parkinson's disease, kidney disease, liver disease, and pregnancy.
Zolpidem	Insomnia		10 mg orally at bedtime.	Drowsiness, dizziness, diarrhea, amnesia, lethargy, hallucinations, ataxia, nausea, headache.	Does not depress ventilation at high altitude. Use as a substitute for temazepam.	Avoid in children, those who are breast-feeding, the elderly, and those with hepatic disease, major depression, pulmonary disease, respiratory depression, and suicidal ideation.
Temazepam	Insomnia		10 mg orally at bedtime	Drowsiness, dizziness, fatigue, ataxia, headache, lethargy, euphoria, amnesia.	Used by the U.S. Air Force in pilots.	Avoid in Soldiers with respiratory depression, hepatic and renal deficiencies, sleep apnea, severe depression, and myasthenia gravis.
Ciprofloxacin	Bacterial diarrhea		500 mg b.i.d. for 5–7 days.	Nausea, vomiting, stomach pain, diarrhea, allergic reaction, rash, tendon rupture.	Drink plenty of fluids while taking the medication.	Do not take with dairy products, antacids, or caffeine. Concurrent administration with tizanidine, or theophylline. Enhances effects of warfarin (anticoagulant).
Metronidazole	Protozoal diarrhea		500 mg three times daily (t.i.d.) for 3 days.	Nausea, diarrhea, headache, loss of appetite, metallic taste, rash.	AVOID ALCOHOL for 3 days after stopping medication.	Enhances effect of warfarin.
Loperamide	Abdominal cramping		4 mg followed by 2 mg after every loose stool.	Constipation, dizziness.		Abdominal pain in the absence of diarrhea, bloody stools, high fever.
Heparin	Thromboembolic event		5,000 units every 8–12 hrs (subcutaneous).	Nosebleed, unusual bruising/bleeding, bloody vomit, bloody urine/stools, nausea, vomiting.		Severe thrombocytopenia, uncontrolled bleeding conditions.

This page intentionally left blank

APPENDIX F

THE LAKE LOUISE ACUTE MOUNTAIN SICKNESS SCORING SYSTEM

Name_____ Age _____ Sex_____ Date _____

Time   ____ ____ ____ ____ ____

Altitude   ____ ____ ____ ____ ____

Self-Reported Symptoms:

1. **Headache:**

No headache	0	____ ____ ____ ____ ____
Mild headache	1	____ ____ ____ ____ ____
Moderate headache	2	____ ____ ____ ____ ____
Severe, incapacitating	3	____ ____ ____ ____ ____

2. **Gastrointestinal:**

No gastrointestinal symptoms	0	____ ____ ____ ____ ____
Poor appetite or nausea	1	____ ____ ____ ____ ____
Moderate nausea or vomiting	2	____ ____ ____ ____ ____
Severe nausea and vomiting, incapacitating	3	____ ____ ____ ____ ____

3. **Fatigue/weakness:**

Not tired or weak	0	____ ____ ____ ____ ____
Mild fatigue/weakness	1	____ ____ ____ ____ ____
Moderate fatigue/weakness	2	____ ____ ____ ____ ____
Severe fatigue/weakness, incapacitating	3	____ ____ ____ ____ ____

4. **Dizzy/lightheaded:**

Not dizzy	0	____ ____ ____ ____ ____
Mild dizziness	1	____ ____ ____ ____ ____
Moderate dizziness	2	____ ____ ____ ____ ____
Severe, incapacitating	3	____ ____ ____ ____ ____

5. **Difficulty sleeping:**

Slept well as usual	0	____ ____ ____ ____ ____
Did not sleep as well as usual	1	____ ____ ____ ____ ____
Woke many times, poor night's sleep	2	____ ____ ____ ____ ____
Could not sleep at all	3	____ ____ ____ ____ ____

Self-Reported Symptom Score: ____ ____ ____ ____

Clinical Assessment:

6. **Change in mental status:**

No change	0	____ ____ ____ ____ ____
Lethargy/lassitude	1	____ ____ ____ ____ ____
Disoriented/confused	2	____ ____ ____ ____ ____
Stupor/semiconsciousness	3	____ ____ ____ ____ ____

7. **Ataxia (heel-to-toe walking):**

No ataxia	0	____ ____ ____ ____ ____
Maneuvers to maintain balance	1	____ ____ ____ ____ ____
Steps off line	2	____ ____ ____ ____ ____
Falls down	3	____ ____ ____ ____ ____
Cannot stand	4	____ ____ ____ ____ ____

8. **Peripheral edema:**

No edema	0	____ ____ ____ ____ ____
One location	1	____ ____ ____ ____ ____
Two or more locations	2	____ ____ ____ ____ ____

Clinical Assessment Score: ____ ____ ____ ____

Total Score (Add Self-Reported Symptom and Clinical Assessment Scores):   ____ ____ ____ ____ ____

This page intentionally left blank

APPENDIX G

HYPERBARIC BAG TREATMENT

G–1. Bag description
There are several models of portable hyperbaric chambers available. Illustrated in Figure G-1 is one model, the Gamow® Bag (NSN: 6515-01-504-6306), available from Chinook Medical Gear, Inc. (http://www.Chinookmed.com). The bag is constructed of durable nylon and reinforced with circular nylon straps. A lengthwise zipper permits easy access and egress for the Soldier, and four clear windows allow visual contact. The bag is pressurized with ambient air to 2 psi by use of a foot pump. (Gamow® is a registered trademark of Portable Hyperbaric, Inc., Illion, New York.)

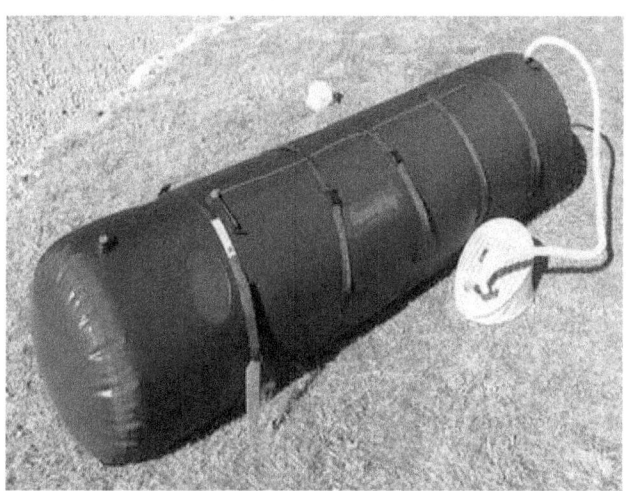

Figure G-1. Gamow® Bag, hyperbaric chamber, Government model

G–2. Treatment
For all portable hyperbaric bags the usual treatment protocol is to place the Soldier into the bag, pump the bag up until the pressure-relief valve hisses, then keep the pressure up by occasional pumping for the duration of the treatment. Continuous pumping is required to ventilate the bag and remove CO_2. Hyperbaric bag treatment durations are generally 2 to 4 hrs for AMS, 4 hrs for HAPE, and 6 hrs for HACE. Maximum therapeutic treatment is obtained by adding supplemental oxygen by nasal cannula or mask with the hyperbaric treatments. Hyperbaric bag treatments can be repeated as necessary until the Soldier clinically improves or is able to descend.

G–3. Precautions
To avoid causing the Soldier to develop barotrauma in the ears or sinuses, compression and decompression of the hyperbaric bag should be done slowly. In cold temperatures, Soldiers should be placed in a sleeping bag within the hyperbaric bag. Conversely, the bag should be shielded from the sun to avoid overheating the Soldier.

This page intentionally left blank

APPENDIX H

HIGH ALTITUDE DEPLOYMENT TIPS

H–1. Prevention categories

Preventing altitude injuries depends on several factors, including prior high altitude experience; proper use of clothing, equipment, and supplies; and appropriate planning for all operational scenarios. In addition to implementing these measures, Soldiers must be carefully observed for signs of distress at altitude and monitored for development of altitude illness. Clothing, shelter, nutrition, and rest/work cycles must be adjusted according to observations.

H–2. Weak link rule

When the first altitude casualty occurs, assess the status of the whole unit.

H–3. Prior high altitude experience

a. Classroom training is not sufficient preparation for altitude deployment; Soldiers must learn to work at altitude before deployment to altitude regions.

b. Training exercises at altitude must initially be conducted for short periods under very controlled conditions and progressively increase in duration and intensity to several days of mission-related tasks under supervision.

c. Training sessions should be designed to provide practical experience under altitude conditions in the following: proper use of altitude equipment during both work and rest periods, efficient shelter construction, meal preparation, and use of other mission-related equipment which may function differently at altitude. Soldiers must be able to complete these tasks efficiently even when at altitude and fatigued.

(1) Soldiers with prior altitude experience will have a better understanding of their own performance at high altitude, and be more efficient at conducting tasks at altitude.

(2) Leadership will gain a better understanding of the capabilities of the unit and the function of equipment at altitude.

H–4. Clothing, equipment, and first aid supplies

a. Soldiers must have access to proper altitude clothing, including items such as silk balaclavas, hiking boots, goggles, sunglasses, Gore-Tex® rain gear, back-up glasses for contact wearers, wicking undergarments, and several changes of socks. (Gore-Tex® is a registered trademark of W.L. Gore & Associates, Inc., Newark, Delaware.)

b. Equipment such as a supplemental oxygen tank, pulse oximeter, i-STAT® blood analyzer, ophthalmoscope, Gamow® Bag, hiking stick, crampon, ice ax, and tent should be tested in a high altitude environment and be usable by Soldiers with reduced manual dexterity due to wearing gloves. (i-STAT® is a registered trademark of i-STAT Corporation, East Princeton, New Jersey.)

c. Medical supplies for a first-aid kit should include but not be limited to the following:

(1) Non-narcotic pain relievers (that is, aspirin, acetaminophen).

(2) Anti-inflammatories (that is, ibuprofen).

(3) Hard candies, throat lozenges, cough suppressant, and decongestant nasal spray.

(4) Sunscreen (SPF 15), zinc oxide, and lip protection.

(5) Minor wound care supplies, Betadine® or iodine-type disinfectant solution, Band-Aids®, moleskin, tape, non-stick bandages, antibiotic ointment, cold compresses, and insect repellent. (Betadine® is a registered trademark of Purdue Frederick Company, Norwalk, Connecticut; Band-Aid® is a registered trademark of Johnson and Johnson Corporation, New Brunswick, New Jersey.)

(6) Iodine tablets (Globaline™, Emergency Drinking Water Germicidal Tablets™ (EDWGT)). (Globaline™ is a trademark of Wisconsin Pharmacal Company, Jackson, Wisconsin; Emergency Drinking Water Germicidal Tablets™ is a trademark of Coghlan's Ltd., Winnipeg, Canada.)

(7) Acute mountain sickness and HACE prophylaxis (that is, acetazolamide and dexamethasone).

(8) High altitude pulmonary edema prophylaxis (that is, nifedipine, tadalafil, salmeterol).

(9) Water-retention medications (furosemide).

(10) Blood-clotting treatment (low-dose subcutaneous heparin).

(11) Malaria prophylaxis (chloroquine, mefloquine).

(12) Anti-diarrheal medication (that is, ciprofloxacin, metronidazole).

(13) Anti-motility medications (loperamide).

(14) Hemorrhoid/constipation medication (Preparation H®, mineral oil). (Preparation H® is a registered trademark of American Home Products, Madison, New Jersey.)

(15) Nausea/vomiting prophylaxis (that is, prochlorperazine).

(16) Insomnia prophylaxis (that is, zolpidem, acetazolamide, temazepam).

(17) Antacids, antioxidant vitamins, One-A-Day® Plus Iron vitamins. (One-A-Day® is a registered trademark of the Bayer Corporation, Pittsburgh, Pennsylvania.)

(18) Oral rehydration solution (available in small packets).

(19) Personal medications for preexisting problems.

H–5. Operational planning
Everything takes longer in an altitude environment, and this may be exacerbated by fatigued Soldiers, poor weather conditions, and exposure that is worse than expected. The weather, unit fitness, work/rest cycles, shelter and nutrition need to be considered during planning.

  a. Weather.

  (1) A reliable source for evaluating elevation, cold stress, and heat stress is necessary. Any altimeter and weather-monitoring devices relied on must be tested in the altitude environment to ensure proper functioning.

  (2) Weather patterns may change abruptly; therefore planning must include contingencies for greater-than-expected exposure to cold or hot conditions.

  (3) Precipitation, winds, and thunderstorms in the mountain environment greatly increase the risk of altitude injury. Careful planning for avoiding these conditions and providing emergency evacuation are imperative.

b. Unit fitness.

(1) Altitude operations may be more physically demanding because of heavier loads (that is, more clothing, oxygen tanks, pulse oximeter, Gamow® Bags), walking on steep and rugged terrain, and less availability of oxygen to the body.

(2) Tired Soldiers are more prone to injury and are less efficient at preparing shelter and meals, which could increase their exposure and risk of injury.

c. Work/rest cycles.

(1) The concept of work/rest cycles can be implemented to avoid excessive energy depletion, fatigue, overheating and sweating in Soldiers who are physically active and to avoid excessive cooling in Soldiers who are immobile.

(2) Sweat accumulation can increase body cooling. Soldiers who have worked hard and have damp clothing must change into dry clothing as soon as possible.

(3) Immobile Soldiers must be aware of extremity cooling. Placing extra insulation on the ground will limit conductive heat loss. Even small movements (stamping feet, swinging arms) will provide some internal heat.

(4) Both wind and solar load affect body temperature and are to be used to advantage. For example, an immobile Soldier positioned out of the wind and exposed to the sun will be much warmer than one who is in the shade and exposed to wind.

d. Shelter.

(1) Adequate shelter is imperative to allow Soldiers to rewarm and dry clothing.

(2) Soldiers must be able to erect shelters in adverse conditions while wearing gloves.

(3) Safety guidelines for use of external heat sources must be followed.

(4) Safety guidelines for locations of camps away from possible lightning strike areas must be followed.

e. Nutrition.

(1) Fluid intake is greatest at mealtime. Providing time for meals will ensure proper hydration as well as energy intake.

(2) Warm meals are important for improving morale and will help rewarm Soldiers who feel cold. Soups are an excellent source of nutrition and hydration.

(3) Tired Soldiers may skip meals to avoid having to prepare stoves and heat water, but this practice will make them more susceptible to high altitude injury and further fatigue.

(4) Eat small meals five to seven times a day.

(5) Eat higher caloric intake meals (that is, First Strike Ration™) to compensate for the extra calories burned in the altitude environment.

(6) Extra precautions are necessary to prevent water supplies from freezing in cold weather.

(7) Hydration of Soldiers can be monitored by noting the color and volume of urine. Dark yellow urine and infrequent urination indicate fluid intake must increase.

This page intentionally left blank

www.ingramcontent.com/pod-product-compliance
Lightning Source LLC
Chambersburg PA
CBHW080706190526
45169CB00006B/2268